SOMATIC YOGA

FOR BEGINNERS

JULIAN APPLE

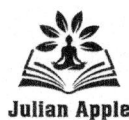

Julian Apple
YOGA & WELLNESS

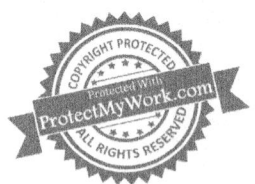

© Copyright 2024 by RMC Publishers - All rights reserved.

This document is geared towards providing exact and reliable information in regard to the topic and issue covered. The publication is sold with the idea that the publisher is not required to render accounting, officially permitted, or otherwise, qualified services. If advice is necessary, legal or professional, a practiced individual in the profession should be ordered.

From a Declaration of Principles which was accepted and approved equally by a Committee of the American Bar Association and a Committee of Publishers and Associations. In no way is it legal to reproduce, duplicate, or transmit any part of this document in either electronic means or in printed format. Recording of this publication is strictly prohibited, and any storage of this document is not allowed unless with written permission from the publisher. All rights reserved.

The information provided herein is stated to be truthful and consistent, in that any liability, in terms of inattention or otherwise, by any usage or abuse of any policies, processes, or directions contained within is the solitary and utter responsibility of the recipient reader. Under no circumstances will any legal responsibility or blame be held against the publisher for any reparation, damages, or monetary loss due to the information herein, either directly or indirectly.

Respective authors own all copyrights not held by the publisher. The information herein is offered for informational purposes solely and is universal as such. The presentation of the information is without a contract or any type of guaranteed assurance. The trademarks that are used are without any consent, and the publication of the trademark is without permission or backing by the trademark owner. All trademarks and brands within this book are for clarifying purposes only and are owned by the owners themselves, not affiliated with this document.

TABLE OF CONTENTS

IIntroduction vii

Chapter 1

Understanding Somatic Yoga 1
    Mindfulness: The foundation of presence 1
    Body awareness: Listening to your inner wisdom 1
    Gentle movement: Nurturing through Motion 2
    Integrating Somatic Principles Into Your Daily Life 2
  The Benefits of Somatic Yoga for Stress and Anxiety. 3
    Stress management through somatic practice 3
    Anxiety relief: Finding calm in the storm. 3
    Overcoming Past Traumas. 3
    How Somatic Yoga Differs from Traditional Yoga 4
    Unique aspects of somatic yoga 5
  The Science Behind Somatic Yoga. 5
   Physiological and Psychological Effects 5
   Research Studies and Expert Opinions 6

Chapter 2

Getting Started with Somatic Yoga. 9
  Preparing Your Space and Mind 9
  Selecting Your Practice Area 9
  Organizing Your Space 9
  Preparing Your Mind 9
  Essential Equipment and Attire. 10
  Choosing Your Mat 10
  Selecting Props 12
    Blocks 12
    Blankets 13
  Comfortable Clothing 15
  Setting Realistic Goals. 17
  The Importance of Realistic Goals. 17
    Goal-Setting Process
. . . . 17
    Examples of Realistic Goals 17
    Tracking Progress 18

Adjusting Goals 18

Chapter 3:

Somatic Yoga Routines for Stress Management, Anxiety Relief, and Overcoming Trauma 19
- Somatic Yoga Poses 19
  - Warm-Up Movements 20
    - Cat-Cow Pose (Marjaryasana-Bitilasana) 20
    - Dynamic Child's Pose (Balasana) 21
    - Spinal Rolls 22
    - Pelvic Tilts 23
    - Gentle Neck Rolls 24
  - Core Somatic Yoga Poses 25
    - Arch and Flatten 25
    - Chair Pose with Arm Waves 26
    - Child's Pose with Arm Walks 27
    - Constructive Rest Position 28
    - Dynamic Bridge Pose 29
    - Dynamic Downward Dog 30
    - Dynamic Tree Pose 31
    - Dynamic Warrior I 32
    - Gentle Fish Pose (Matsyasana) 33
    - Knees to Chest Rocking 35
    - Leg Slides 36
    - Lying Hip Release 37
    - Pelvic Clock 38
    - Quadruped Cat Stretch 39
    - Reclined Butterfly Pose 40
    - Reclined Hamstring Stretch 41
    - Reclined Spinal Twist 42
    - Seated Arm Circles 43
    - Seated Cat-Cow 44
    - Seated Figure Four Stretch 45
    - Seated Forward Fold with Rocking 46
    - Seated Side Bend 47
    - Side-Lying Leg Lifts 48
    - Somatic Bridge Pose 49
    - Somatic Chest Opener 50
    - Somatic Cobra Pose 51
    - Somatic Crescent Lunge 52
    - Somatic Forward Fold 53

- Somatic Frog Pose ... 54
- Somatic Half-Bow Pose ... 55
- Somatic Hip Rolls ... 56
- Standing Pelvic Tilts ... 57
- Somatic Pigeon Pose ... 58
- Somatic Plank Pose ... 59
- Somatic Scapula Mobilization ... 60
- Somatic Seated Twist ... 61
- Somatic Side Stretch ... 62
- Somatic Shoulder Bridge ... 63
- Somatic Shoulder Shrugs ... 64
- Somatic Sunbird Pose ... 65
- Somatic Twists ... 66
- Somatic Tabletop Cat-Cow ... 67
- Somatic Warrior II ... 68
- Somatic Wave ... 69
- Sphinx Pose ... 70
- Standing Forward Bend with Swaying ... 71
- Supine Arm Circles ... 72
- Supine PSOAS Release ... 73
- Tabletop Arm and Leg Extensions ... 74
- Cool-Down Movements ... 75
  - Supine Knee-to-Chest Pose ... 75
  - Legs Up the Wall Pose/Waterfall pose ... 76
  - Supine One-Legged Twist ... 77
  - Corpse Pose (Savasana) ... 78
  - Guided Body Scan with Flex and Relax ... 79
- Access to Your Gifts ... 81
- Routine 1: Quick Stress-Relief (10-15 minutes) ... 82
- Routine 2: Anxiety-Calming Practice (20-30 minutes) ... 82
- Routine 3: Trauma-Informed Practice (30-40 minutes) ... 83
- Routine 4: Morning Energizer (15-20 minutes) ... 83
- Routine 5: Evening Wind-Down (25-30 minutes) ... 84
- General tips for proper form and alignment ... 85

Chapter 4

Managing Anxiety with Somatic Yoga ... 87
- Understanding Anxiety and Its Triggers ... 87
- Somatic Yoga Poses for Anxiety Relief ... 89
- Breathing Techniques for Anxiety Management ... 93
  - Square Breathing ... 93

       4-7-8 Breath 93
       Belly Breathing 93

Chapter 5

Stress Relief Through Somatic Yoga 95
   Identifying Stressors in Your Life...................................95
   Somatic Yoga for Relaxation......................................96
   Meditation and Mindfulness Practices
       Meditation Technique: Body Scan Meditation 98
       Mindfulness Exercise: STOP Technique......................99

Chapter 6

Trauma Release with Somatic Yoga................................101
   Routine 101
   Additional Somatic Practices for Trauma Release 103

Chapter 7

28-Day Somatic Yoga Plan......................................105
   Routines and techniques 105
       Anxiety Relief Routine (15-20 minutes) 105
       Stress Relief Routine (15-20 minutes) 106
       Trauma Release Routine (15 to 20 minutes) 107
       Breathing Techniques 107
       Mindfulness Practices 108
   28-Day Plan 109
       Week 1: Foundation 109
       Week 2: Building Awareness...............................110
       Week 3: Deepening Practice 111
       Week 4: Integration......................................112

Conclusion: Maintaining Your Somatic Yoga Practice 115
   Continuing Your Journey 115
   Adapting to Life Changes......................................116
   Strategies for Staying Engaged 116

Exercise List..119

References 121

INTRODUCTION

Modern living is filled with stress and anxiety, and the lingering effects of past traumas have become way too common. Many of us find ourselves caught in a cycle of tension and unease, searching for effective ways to find balance and peace in our daily lives. If you have picked up this book, chances are you are one of the many individuals seeking a holistic, long-term approach to overcoming these challenges.

Somatic yoga is grounded on the belief that your body holds the key to your emotional and mental well-being. Learning to listen to and work with your body can help you heal and become more resilient to life's challenges.

Somatic Yoga for Beginners has been designed to help you discover somatic yoga, a powerful practice that focuses on the intricate connection between your mind and body. Unlike traditional yoga forms that center on physical postures, somatic yoga addresses the root causes of stress, anxiety, and trauma stored within your body. This approach helps you to find both temporary relief as well as a lasting transformation.

While reading Somatic Yoga for Beginners you will discover sustainable, low-impact routines that are flexible and adaptable to your busy schedule. The somatic yoga practices presented are gentle yet effective, making them suitable for all fitness levels and even those with previous injuries.

In addition, you will learn:

- Practical knowledge on incorporating somatic yoga into your daily life.
- Detailed routines designed for stress relief, anxiety management, and trauma release.
- Expert advice backed by scientific research.
- And so much more.

This book focuses on you, allowing you to step away from the constant stressors of life for a moment so that you can rebalance, refocus, and gradually begin to release the stored trauma within you.

SOMATIC YOGA FOR WEIGHT LOSS

We recognize that maintaining a reduced-stress lifestyle amidst the chaos of daily life is a significant challenge. That is why we have created a 28-day program that gradually introduces you to the principles and practices of somatic yoga. By the end of this journey, you will have the tools and knowledge to continue your practice independently, creating a sustainable path to lasting joy and inner peace.

Here are the key themes that we will explore throughout this book and that are fundamental to the practice of somatic yoga and its benefits for stress, anxiety, and trauma.

1. Mind-body connection: Harnessing the intricate relationship between your thoughts, emotions, and physical sensations is essential.
2. Embodied awareness: Techniques to develop a deeper sense of awareness within your body will enable you to identify and release areas of tension and stored stress.
3. Gentle movement and breath work: Soft, flowing movements and breathing exercises form the core of somatic yoga practice.
4. Neuroplasticity and healing: Discover how somatic yoga can help rewire your nervous system, promoting resilience and recovery from stress and trauma.
5. Mindfulness and present-moment awareness: Learn how to cultivate a state of mindful presence, reducing anxiety about the future and regrets about the past.
6. Self-regulation techniques: We will teach you powerful tools to manage your emotional state and stress levels independently.
7. Integration into daily life: You will learn how to incorporate somatic principles into your everyday activities, not just during dedicated practice time.
8. Sustainable wellness: We focus on creating lasting change through consistent, manageable practices rather than quick fixes.
9. Empowerment and self-discovery: Throughout your journey, you will be encouraged to listen to your own body's wisdom and become your own best teacher.

Keep in mind that change takes time and patience. Be kind to yourself, listen to your body, and trust the process. Welcome to the world of somatic yoga—Your 28-day Transformative Journey to Turn Trauma and Anxiety into Lasting Joy. - your path to turning trauma and anxiety into lasting joy begins here. Let's take the first step together towards a calmer, more centered you.

Chapter 1

UNDERSTANDING SOMATIC YOGA

Somatic yoga is founded on three interlinked principles: mindfulness, body awareness, and gentle movement. These tenets work in harmony to create a powerful practice that can transform your relationship with your body and mind.

Mindfulness: The foundation of presence

Mindfulness is the art of being fully grounded in the present moment, without judgment. In somatic yoga, this extends beyond pure mental awareness—it is about tuning into your entire being. As you practice, you will learn to observe your thoughts, emotions, and physical sensations with curiosity and compassion.

To try full-body mindfulness, try closing your eyes and taking a deep breath. Notice the sensation of the air entering your nostrils, filling your lungs, and then leaving your body. This simple act of "noticing" is mindfulness in action.

Body awareness: Listening to your inner wisdom

Body awareness, or interoception, is your ability to sense and understand the signals your body sends you. Many of us have learned to ignore these signals, pushing ourselves through discomfort or stress. Somatic yoga helps you reconnect with your body's innate wisdom.

As you develop body awareness, you might notice:

- Areas of tension or pain.
- Emotional responses that manifest physically (like a tight chest when anxious).

- Subtle shifts in your energy levels throughout the day.

Gentle movement: Nurturing through Motion

Gentle movement forms the physical component of somatic yoga. Unlike more vigorous forms of exercise, these soft, flowing movements are designed to release tension and stress, improve flexibility, and promote relaxation. In moving slowly and mindfully, you give your body and mind the opportunity to fully process each movement and its effects.

Here is a simple somatic movement you can try before beginning with the exercises in this book.

- Slowly roll your shoulders forward, up, back, and down. Pay attention to any sensations—perhaps a subtle stretch or release of tension. This is the essence of gentle, mindful movement in somatic yoga.

Integrating Somatic Principles Into Your Daily Life

These principles intertwine to create a practice that nurtures both your physical and mental well-being. For instance, as you move through a gentle stretching sequence, you will simultaneously practice mindfulness by focusing on your breath and body awareness by tuning into the sensations in your muscles and joints.

The beauty of somatic yoga lies in its applicability to everyday life. Here are some ways to incorporate these principles beyond your formal practice:

- **Start your day with a body scan**: Lying in bed, mentally scan your body from head to toe, noticing any areas of tension or discomfort.
- **Practice mindful eating**: Pay attention to the flavors, textures, and sensations of each bite.
- **Take movement breaks**: Set reminders to do gentle stretches or movements throughout your workday.
- **End your day with reflection**: Before sleep, check in with your body and mind, acknowledging how you feel without judgment.

The Benefits of Somatic Yoga for Stress and Anxiety

Somatic yoga offers a powerful toolkit for managing stress and anxiety in our fast-paced world. By focusing on the mind-body connection, this practice helps you develop resilience and find inner calm, even in the most challenging situations.

Stress management through somatic practice

Stress often manifests through physical signs including tense shoulders, clenched jaw, or an upset stomach. Somatic yoga teaches you how to spot these stress symptoms quickly, enabling you to address stress before it overwhelms you.

Gentle movements and breathwork will help you manage stress by:

- Activating the parasympathetic nervous system (rest and digest system), triggering the relaxation response.
- Teaching you to release physical tension through gentle movement.
- Improving your ability to stay grounded in the present moment, rather than worrying about the future.

Anxiety relief: Finding calm in the storm

For those struggling with anxiety, somatic yoga can be a powerful tool for finding inner peace by:

- Teaching you to recognize the physical sensations of anxiety in your body.
- Providing techniques to regulate your breath, which can quickly calm an anxious mind.
- Improving your ability to sit with uncomfortable sensations without becoming overwhelmed.

Overcoming Past Traumas

Trauma often leaves imprints not just in our minds, but also in our bodies. It may manifest as chronic tension or physical discomfort or full physical responses like panic attacks or reliving the trauma itself. Somatic yoga offers a gentle path toward healing. Through mindful movement and body awareness, you can safely explore these sensations, gradually releasing stored trauma and finding relief.

Key Benefits Summary

The practice of somatic yoga offers you benefits beyond stress and anxiety management. Here is a non-exhaustive list of these benefits:

- Improved body awareness (enabling you to recognize and address stress early).
- Enhanced relaxation response (helping you find calm more easily).
- Enhanced emotional regulation (giving you more control over your reactions).
- Improved sleep quality (crucial for overall mental health).
- Increased resilience to daily stressors.
- Greater self-awareness and self-acceptance.
- A sense of empowerment in your healing journey.
- Better overall physical health, including reduced chronic pain.
- A sense of empowerment in your healing journey.

How Somatic Yoga Differs from Traditional Yoga

While somatic yoga shares some similarities with traditional yoga practices, it offers a unique approach that sets it apart. Traditional yoga often focuses on achieving specific postures or sequences and emphasizes physical alignment and strength. Somatic yoga, on the other hand, prioritizes the internal experience of movement and sensation.

In a traditional yoga class, you might be guided through a series of poses, holding each for a set time. In contrast, a somatic yoga session invites you to explore gentle, fluid movements, paying close attention to how each movement feels in your body. There's less emphasis on "correct" form and more on what feels right for your unique body.

Another key difference lies in the pace. Traditional yoga can sometimes be quite vigorous, especially in styles like Vinyasa or Ashtanga. Somatic yoga is intentionally slow and gentle, allowing time for deep awareness and integration of the mind-body connection.

Unique aspects of somatic yoga

- Emphasis on sensation: Rather than aiming for a particular shape, somatic yoga invites you to explore how movements feel in your body.
- Individualized practice: There's no "one-size-fits-all" in somatic yoga. You are encouraged to adapt the movements to suit your own body's needs.
- Integration of neuroscience: Somatic yoga incorporates an understanding of the nervous system and how movement affects our mental state.

The significance of these differences becomes clear when we consider the goals of somatic yoga. While traditional yoga can certainly be relaxing and stress-reducing, somatic yoga is specifically designed to release deeply held tensions and trauma. Its gentle approach makes it accessible to people of all fitness levels or with physical limitations or injuries.

While both somatic and traditional yoga can be beneficial, they have distinct approaches and focuses.

The unique approach of somatic yoga makes it:

- Accessible to people of all fitness levels and abilities.
- Particularly beneficial for those dealing with chronic pain, injuries, or trauma.
- Effective for developing a deeper mind-body connection.

The Science Behind Somatic Yoga

The effectiveness of somatic yoga is supported by a growing body of scientific research. At its core, somatic yoga works by influencing the nervous system, particularly the autonomic nervous system which controls our stress response.

When we experience stress or trauma, our sympathetic nervous system—responsible for the "fight-or-flight" response—becomes overactive. Somatic yoga helps to activate the parasympathetic nervous system, often called the "rest and digest" system. This shift promotes relaxation, reduces anxiety, and supports overall well-being.

Physiological and Psychological Effects

Somatic yoga influences multiple systems in the body:

- **Nervous System**: It helps balance the autonomic nervous system, reducing the dominance of the "fight or flight" response.
- **Endocrine System**: Practice can help regulate stress hormones like cortisol which is called "the stress hormone".
- **Musculoskeletal System**: Gentle movements can improve flexibility and reduce chronic tension.
- **Brain**: Mindfulness practices have been shown to change brain structure, particularly in areas related to emotional regulation and self-awareness.

Research Studies and Expert Opinions

While research specifically on somatic yoga is still emerging, studies on similar mind-body practices provide strong support for its potential benefits:

- A study published in the Journal of Traumatic Stress found that body-oriented interventions significantly reduced symptoms of PTSD in trauma survivors (van de Kamp., et al. 2023).
- Research published in Scientific Reports showed that slow, mindful movement combined with breath awareness led to reduced cortisol levels and improved mood (Fincham et al., 2023).
- A study published in Psychology and Neuroscience highlighted how interoceptive practices (like those used in somatic yoga) can improve emotional regulation and reduce anxiety (Menezes et al., 2015).

Neuroimaging studies have also provided insights into how these practices affect the brain. Research has shown that mindfulness practices can lead to changes in brain structure, particularly in areas associated with emotional regulation and self-awareness.

While more research specific to somatic yoga is needed, the existing evidence strongly supports its potential benefits for stress, anxiety, and trauma. As you embark on your somatic yoga journey, you can feel confident that you are engaging in a practice grounded in a scientific understanding of the mind-body connection.

Remember, everyone's experience is unique, and the most important thing is to approach your practice with curiosity and compassion for yourself.

CHAPTER 2

GETTING STARTED WITH SOMATIC YOGA

Embarking on your somatic yoga journey is an exciting step towards improved well-being. This chapter will guide you through the essential preparations, equipping you with the knowledge to create an ideal practice environment, choose appropriate gear, and set achievable goals. Let's begin this transformative path together.

Preparing Your Space and Mind

Creating a nurturing environment is crucial for a fulfilling somatic yoga practice. Your space should invite calm and focus, allowing you to tune into your body's subtle signals.

Selecting Your Practice Area

Choose a quiet spot in your home where you feel at ease. This could be a corner of your bedroom, a spare room, or even a peaceful outdoor area. Ensure the space is free from clutter and distractions.

Organizing Your Space

Arrange your area to promote a sense of order and tranquility. Keep your yoga mat and props easily accessible. Consider incorporating elements that soothe your senses —perhaps a small plant, a calming image, or a soft light source.

Preparing Your Mind

Before beginning your practice, take a moment to center yourself. Try this simple relaxation technique:

1. Sit or lie comfortably.
2. Close your eyes and take three deep breaths.
3. Scan your body from head to toe, noticing any areas of tension.
4. Set an intention for your practice, such as "I am open to listening to my body."

This brief ritual helps transition your mind from daily concerns to the present moment, enhancing your somatic yoga experience.

Essential Equipment and Attire

While somatic yoga requires minimal equipment, a few key items can greatly enhance your practice.

1. **Yoga mat**: Provides cushioning and defines your practice space.
2. **Comfortable clothing**: Allows free movement and body awareness.
3. **Blanket or towel**: Offers extra support and warmth.
4. **Yoga blocks**: Assists in maintaining proper alignment.
5. **Bolster or firm pillow**: Supports restorative poses.

Choosing Your Mat

When selecting a mat for the practice of somatic yoga, you must take various factors into account. If you have sensitive joints, consider a thicker mat for extra comfort. Eco-friendly options are available for environmentally conscious practitioners.

Here is a list of the most important aspects to consider when choosing your mat:

- **Thickness and cushioning**: Somatic yoga involves gentle, floor-based movements, so a mat with good cushioning (at least 5-6mm thick) can provide the necessary support and comfort.
- **Material**: Look for eco-friendly materials like natural rubber, TPE, or sustainably sourced PVC. These materials tend to be more durable and offer better grip.

- **Texture and grip**: A non-slip surface is crucial to prevent slipping, especially during slow transitions.
- **Durability**: Investing in a high-quality mat ensures it will last longer and maintain its performance over time.
- **Portability**: If you plan to take your mat to classes, you should pay attention to its weight and how easy it will be to carry.

Here are some of the best mats that cater to the needs of somatic yoga practitioners:

Brand	Features	Pros	Cons
Manduka PRO Yoga Mat	High-density cushioning, excellent durability, and a non-slip surface.	Provides superior comfort and joint protection, ideal for slow and mindful movements.	Heavier and requires a break-in period for optimal grip.
Liforme Yoga Mat	Alignment markers, eco-friendly materials, and excellent grip.	The alignment markers help maintain proper posture, and the mat provides a firm yet comfortable surface.	Higher price point and heavier weight.
Jade Yoga Harmony Mat	Made from natural rubber, excellent grip, and comfortable cushioning.	Eco-friendly, offers great traction, and is suitable for various yoga styles.	Slightly heavier and requires regular cleaning to maintain grip.
Hugger Mugger Para Rubber Yoga Mat	Dual-textured surface for grip, eco-friendly, and thick cushioning.	Provides excellent support and comfort, especially for floor-based practices.	Heavier than some other mats and has a natural rubber smell initially.
Gaiam Performance Dry-Grip Yoga Mat	Non-slip surface, lightweight, and durable.	Affordable, easy to transport, and offers good grip even in sweaty conditions.	Less cushioning compared to premium mats.
Alo Yoga Warrior Mat	Dense cushioning, excellent grip, and moisture-wicking properties.	Comfortable and supportive, ideal for both gentle and dynamic practices.	Higher price point and may be heavy for some users.

Choosing the right mat can enhance your somatic yoga practice by providing the necessary comfort and support, allowing you to focus on mindful movement and body awareness.

Selecting Props

Start with basic props like blocks and a blanket. As you advance, you might explore additional props like straps or bolsters.

Blocks

When practicing somatic yoga, having the right blocks can significantly enhance your experience by providing support, stability, and comfort during various poses and movements.

Just as when choosing your mat, some factors are important to consider when choosing your blocks.

- **Material**: Blocks are typically made from foam or cork. Foam blocks are lightweight and softer, while cork blocks are firmer and provide more stability.
- **Size**: Standard yoga blocks are 9" x 6" x 4". Some practitioners prefer when they are larger for better support.
- **Firmness**: Depending on your needs, choose between softer foam blocks for comfort or firmer cork blocks for stability.
- **Weight**: Foam blocks are lighter and easier to transport, while cork blocks are heavier but provide more solid support. If you need to carry your blocks to different locations, lightweight options like the Gaiam foam blocks are convenient.
- **Comfort and support**: Opt for blocks that provide a good balance of softness and support. High-density foam blocks like those from Hugger Mugger or Manduka's recycled foam blocks are excellent choices.
- **Stability**: For poses requiring more stability, cork blocks like those from Manduka or Yoloha are ideal due to their firmness and non-slip properties.
- **Eco-friendliness**: If sustainability is important to you, look for blocks made from recycled materials or sustainable sources like cork.

Here are some of the best blocks that cater to the needs of somatic yoga practitioners:

GETTING STARTED WITH SOMATIC YOGA

Brand	Features	Pros	Cons
Manduka Cork Yoga Block	Made from sustainable cork, firm, and offers excellent grip.	Durable, provides solid support, and eco-friendly.	Heavier than foam blocks.
Gaiam Yoga Block	Made from durable foam, lightweight, and offers a comfortable grip.	Affordable, available in various colors, and easy to transport.	Less firm compared to cork blocks.
Hugger Mugger Foam Yoga Block	High-density foam, soft and supportive, with beveled edges for comfort.	Lightweight, durable, and provides excellent support.	May compress slightly under heavy weight.
Lululemon Lift and Lengthen Yoga Block	Made from high-density foam, firm with a smooth finish.	Provides a stable base, comfortable to use, and is aesthetically pleasing.	Higher price point.
Manduka Recycled Foam Yoga Block	Made from recycled foam, lightweight, and firm.	Eco-friendly, durable, and provides excellent support.	Slightly more expensive than other foam blocks.
Yoloha Cork Yoga Block	Made from sustainable cork, firm, and non-slip surface.	Eco-friendly, provides excellent stability and is lightweight for a cork block.	Can be pricier compared to foam blocks.

Having the right blocks can greatly enhance your somatic yoga practice, providing the necessary support and stability to help you focus on mindful movement and body awareness.

Blankets

Choosing the right blankets for somatic yoga is essential for providing comfort, support, and warmth during your practice.

Here are some of its characteristics you should pay attention to:

- **Material**: Choose between wool, cotton, or synthetic blends. Wool and cotton provide natural warmth and comfort, while synthetic blends offer durability and ease of care.
- **Size and thickness**: Larger and thicker blankets offer better support and can be folded to create different heights for various poses.
- **Durability**: Make sure the blanket is well-made and can withstand regular use and washing.
- **Comfort**: Softness and texture are important for comfort, especially during prolonged poses or relaxation.
- **Eco-friendliness**: Consider blankets made from recycled or organic materials if sustainability is a priority for you.

Here is a selection of blankets that cater to the needs of somatic yoga practitioners:

Brand	Features	Pros	Cons
Manduka Recycled Wool Blanket	Made from a blend of recycled wool and synthetic fibers, soft, and warm.	Provides excellent warmth and comfort, is durable, and is eco-friendly.	Can be a bit heavy for some users.
Hugger Mugger Mexican Yoga Blanket	Made from a blend of cotton, acrylic, and polyester, colorful, and versatile.	Soft, durable, and large enough to fold into different thicknesses for various uses.	Requires washing before first use to soften.
Yoga Accessories Traditional Mexican Yoga Blanket	Made from a blend of acrylic, polyester, and cotton, vibrant colors, and traditional design.	Affordable, versatile, and provides good support and comfort.	May shed initially and requires washing before use.

Brand	Features	Pros	Cons
Barefoot Yoga Co. Deluxe Mexican Yoga Blanket	Made from recycled fibers, tightly woven, and sturdy.	Soft, durable, and provides excellent support and warmth.	Slightly higher price point.
B Yoga B Calm Wool Yoga Blanket	Made from 100% wool, soft, and provides excellent insulation.	Natural material, very warm, and comfortable.	More expensive and requires special care for cleaning.

GETTING STARTED WITH SOMATIC YOGA

| Lotuscrafts Yoga Blanket Savasana | Made from 100% organic cotton, soft, and cozy. | Eco-friendly, breathable, and versatile for various uses in yoga practice. | Less firm compared to wool or thicker blankets. |

Using the right blanket can greatly enhance your somatic yoga practice by providing the necessary support, comfort, and warmth, allowing you to focus on mindful movement and relaxation.

Comfortable Clothing

When it comes to yoga clothing, just like for the rest of your equipment, there are some features you should be careful about.

- Comfort: Look for soft, stretchy, and moisture-wicking fabrics that provide comfort and support during your practice.
- Fit: Make sure that the clothing fits well and allows for a full range of motion without being too tight or restrictive.
- Durability: High-quality materials and construction ensure the clothing lasts through numerous washes and wears.
- Style: Choose designs and colors that make you feel confident and motivated.
- Eco-friendliness: You may also consider brands that use sustainable materials and ethical manufacturing practices.

Therefore, you should opt for breathable, stretchy fabrics that move with your body. Avoid overly loose clothing that might interfere with your awareness of body positioning. Remember, comfort is key - wear what allows you to focus on your practice rather than on your outfit.

Here are some of the top brands known for their high-quality yoga apparel.

Brand	Features	Pros	Cons
Lululemon	High-performance fabrics, stylish designs, and a wide range of options for different body types.	Excellent durability, comfortable fit, and moisture-wicking properties and Durability	Higher price point.

Brand	Features	Pros	Cons
Alo Yoga	Trendy designs, high-quality fabrics, and a focus on both performance and style.	Comfortable and supportive, great for both yoga and casual wear.	Can be expensive.
Athleta	Versatile and stylish clothing, eco-friendly materials, and inclusive sizing.	Durable, comfortable, and suitable for various activities beyond yoga.	Some items can be pricey.
Manduka	High-performance and sustainable materials, simple and functional designs, and a focus on performance.	Eco-friendly, durable, and comfortable.	Limited variety compared to fashion-focused brands.
prAna	Sustainable and ethical manufacturing, versatile designs, and high-quality materials.	Eco-friendly, durable, and comfortable for both yoga and everyday wear.	Some styles may not be as fashion-forward.
Brand	**Features**	**Pros**	**Cons**
Outdoor Voices	Trendy, colorful, and stylish designs, versatile for various activities, and high-quality fabrics.	Comfortable, supportive, and suitable for a range of activities.	Limited options specifically designed for yoga.
Girlfriend Collective	Sustainable and eco-friendly materials, inclusive sizing, and trendy designs.	Comfortable, durable, and made from recycled materials.	Somewhat limited color options.
Beyond Yoga	Soft and luxurious fabrics, inclusive sizing, and stylish designs.	Extremely comfortable, flattering fit, and versatile for various activities.	Can be on the pricier side.

Being well-equipped supports your practice by allowing you to focus on the sensations in your body rather than on discomfort or distractions. However, remember that the most important tool in somatic yoga is your own body awareness.

Setting Realistic Goals

Establishing achievable goals is vital for maintaining motivation and tracking your progress in somatic yoga. Your goals should reflect your personal journey and current capabilities.

The Importance of Realistic Goals

Setting attainable goals helps build confidence and maintains your enthusiasm for the practice. Unrealistic expectations might lead to frustration or disappointment, potentially derailing your somatic yoga journey.

Goal-Setting Process

1. Reflect on your motivations: Why are you drawn to somatic yoga?
2. Assess your current state: Consider your physical condition, time availability, and stress levels.
3. Visualize your desired outcome: What do you hope to achieve through this practice?
4. Break down large goals into smaller ones, measurable steps.
5. Set a timeline: Be generous with yourself, allowing room for adaptation.

Examples of Realistic Goals

- Practice somatic yoga for 15 minutes, three times a week for the first month.
- Master one new somatic movement technique each week.
- Reduce tension in my shoulders by 50% within three months of consistent practice.
- Incorporate a 5-minute body scan into my daily routine.

Tracking Progress

Keep a simple journal of your practice. Note the duration of your training sessions, specific exercises, and any physical or emotional observations. This record will help you spot subtle improvements over time.

Adjusting Goals

Regularly review your goals and adjust them if needed. If you are consistently meeting your targets, consider setting more challenging goals. If you are struggling, it is perfectly acceptable to modify your goals to better suit your current circumstances.

Remember, the journey of somatic yoga is deeply personal. Your goals should reflect your unique needs and aspirations. Be patient and considerate with yourself. Celebrate all the victories along the way, even the smallest. With consistent practice and realistic expectations, you will soon feel the transformative effects of somatic yoga.

CHAPTER 3

SOMATIC YOGA ROUTINES FOR STRESS MANAGEMENT, ANXIETY RELIEF, AND OVERCOMING TRAUMA

In this chapter, we will begin guiding you through practical somatic yoga routines designed to help you manage stress, alleviate anxiety, and work through stored trauma. These gentle, mindful practices are tailored to fit various schedules and can be easily integrated into your daily life. Through these routines, you will begin to unlock a powerful toolkit for cultivating inner calm and resilience.

Somatic Yoga Poses

Before we delve into specific routines, let's familiarize ourselves with some key somatic yoga poses that form the foundation of our stress-relief practices.

Warm-Up Movements

Cat-Cow Pose (Marjaryasana-Bitilasana)

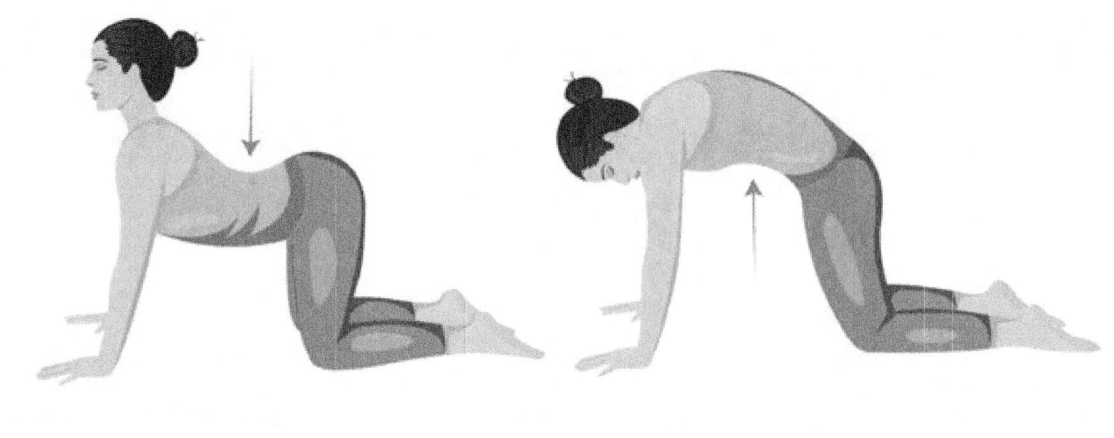

- Begin your workout on your hands and knees with your spine straight and your head in a neutral position. Your neck and spine should form a straight line. This is your tabletop position.
- Inhale deeply while curving your lower back and bringing your head up, tilting your pelvis up. This is your cow position.
- Hold for 2 breath counts.
- On your next exhale, bring your abdomen in, sucking your belly toward your spine, arching your spine, and bringing your head and pelvis down. This is your cat position.
- Hold for 2 breath counts.
- Alternate between cat and cow 5 times.
- Return to your tabletop position.

Dynamic Child's Pose (Balasana)

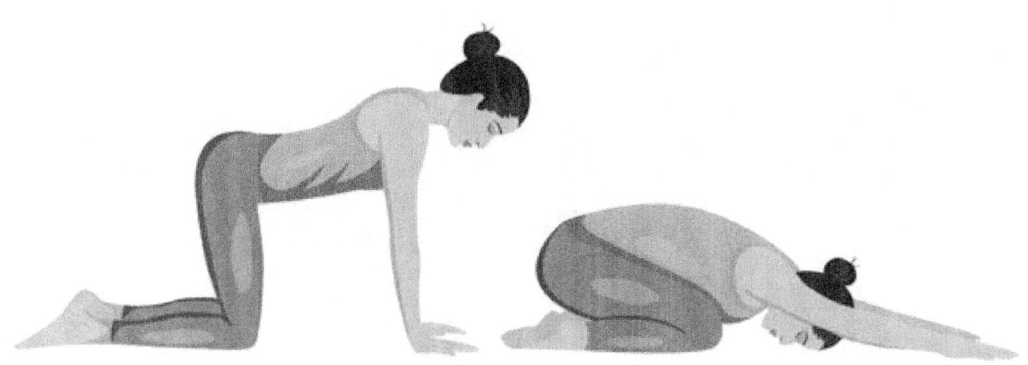

- From your tabletop position, untuck your toes so that the tops of your feet are flat on your mat.
- Exhale deeply and as you do, lower your chest towards your knees and move your hands about a hand-length forward.
- Bring your knees slightly wider than hip-width apart and allow your big toes to touch each other.
- Bring focus to your breath and allow your belly to sink lower between your thighs.
- On your next conscious inhale, push through your thighs, lifting your body back into the tabletop position.
- Bring focus to your breath once more, allowing your body to right itself and stretching your thighs.
- Exhale, and drop back to your child's pose, belly sinking to the mat.
- Repeat this movement 5 times.
- Complete your sequence in a child's pose.

Spinal Rolls

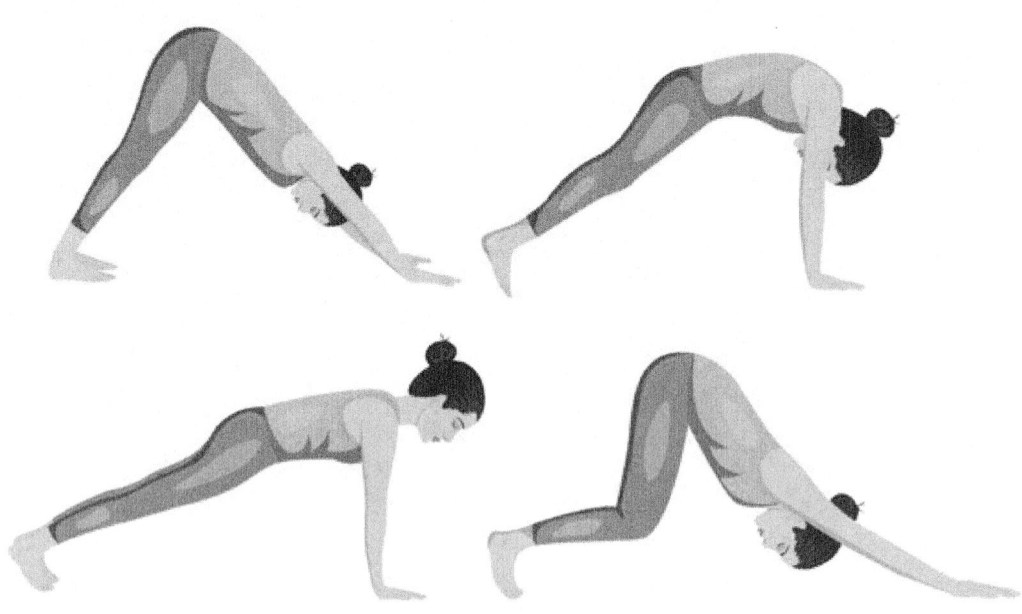

- From your Child's pose, tuck your toes in and push your pelvis up toward the ceiling, straightening your legs so that your body creates a v-shape. This is the downward-facing dog position.
- Bring focus to your breath, and as you exhale, slowly arch your upper back as you begin to lower your pelvis to the mat, entering into a plank position.
- Hold this position for 2 breath counts, focusing on maintaining a straight spine.
- Inhale and bend your knees, as you push your pelvis up toward the ceiling again, entering into the Downward Facing Dog position.
- Flow between Half-Child's Pose, Downward Facing Dog, and Plank Pose 5 times, making sure to focus on your breath.
- To complete your sequence, end in the Half-Child's pose. Lower your knees to the mat to enter into a tabletop position.
- Slide your legs out behind you and carefully roll over into the supine position.

SOMATIC YOGA ROUTINES FOR STRESS MANAGEMENT, ANXIETY RELIEF, AND OVERCOMING TRAUMA

Pelvic Tilts

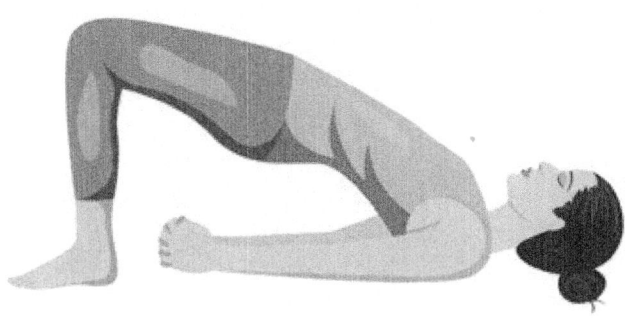

- From your supine position, bend your knees, bringing your ankles toward your behind.
- Bring your hands down to rest on the mat at your sides and in line with your hips.
- Open your feet about hip-width apart.
- Inhale deeply and as you do, push through your feet, lifting your pelvis up toward the ceiling.
- Keep your feet, upper shoulders, and head grounded into the mat.
- Exhale, and if you can, slide your hands under your lifted pelvis, closing them behind you.
- Draw focus to your breath and hold your bridge for 5 breath counts.
- On your 5th count, drop your pelvis very slightly, immediately raising it back to the elevated position. These are micro-movements.
- Complete 10 micromovement tilts before sliding your arms out from under you and lowering your body back to the mat.
- Using your abdominal muscles, come to a comfortable seated position.

SOMATIC YOGA FOR WEIGHT LOSS

Gentle Neck Rolls

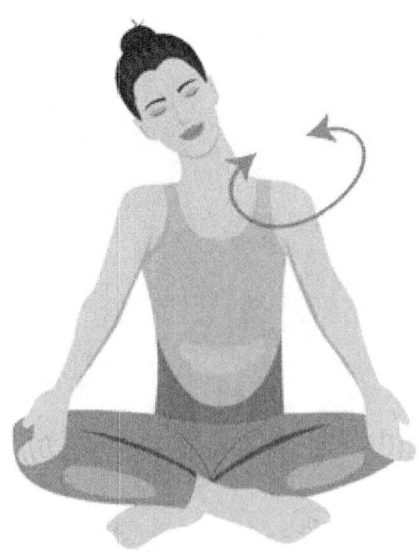

- In your seated position, cross your legs comfortably.
- Rest your hands, palms facing upward on your knees, and arms straightened.
- Lengthen your spine, relax your shoulder, and push your chest out.
- Inhale and begin rolling your neck in a clockwise position first. Be sure to keep your movements controlled and slow.
- Complete 5 neck rolls in the clockwise position and 5 in the anticlockwise position.

These warm-up movements gently awaken the body, promoting circulation and releasing initial tension. They prepare you for deeper work in the core poses.

Core Somatic Yoga Poses

Arch and Flatten

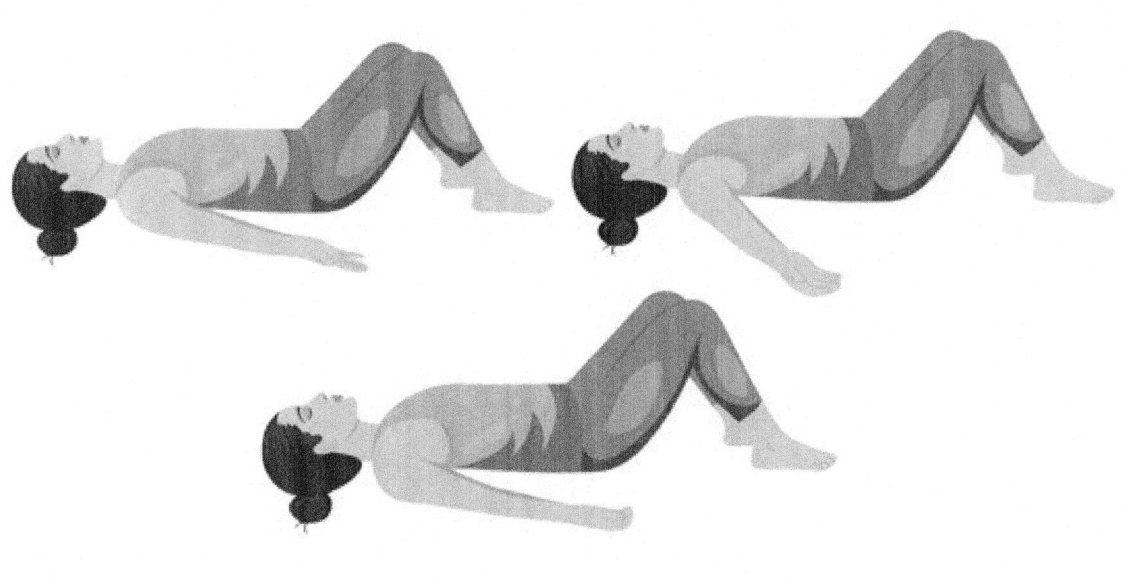

- Begin this sequence by lying flat on your back with your feet on the floor.
- Place your hands on the floor, palms facing up, about a hand's length from your hips.
- Inhale and arch your back slightly, pressing your shoulders into the mat and ensuring your glutes remain grounded.
- Hold for 2 breath counts and release, flattening your back back to the mat.
- On your next inhale, arch your back once more.
- Repeat between your arch and flatten movements 10 times.
- Return to your center by using your abdominal muscles to sit up. Once seated, push up with your arms and legs to a standing position.

SOMATIC YOGA FOR WEIGHT LOSS

Chair Pose with Arm Waves

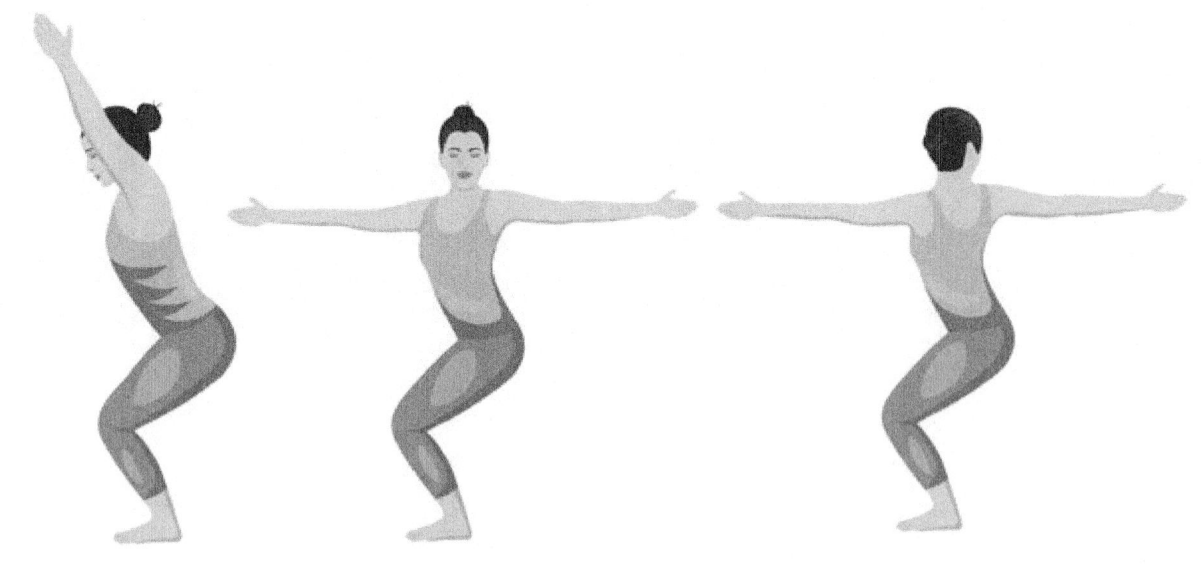

- From a standing position, bring your feet together and root yourself to earth.
- Bend your knees slightly, bringing the weight of your body on the heels of your feet.
- Tuck your pelvis in and lift your ribcage so that your neck is in a neutral position. This is your chair position.
- Inhale deeply, lifting your hands above your head, bringing your palms together in a prayer position.
- Exhale deeply and open your arms, bringing them down to your sides.
- Gently rotate your upper body to the right first and then the left, taking care not to hyperextend your knees.
- Return to your center position.
- Inhale and repeat this pose 5 times.
- To return to your center, inhale deeply and drop your knees to the mat, entering into a child's pose.

Child's Pose with Arm Walks

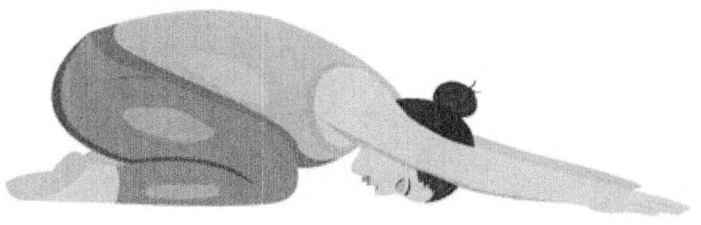

- From a kneeling position, your toes and knees together, rest most of your weight on your heels.
- Place the palms of your hands on the floor and drop your pelvis to the mat, pushing through your knees to form an easy gap.
- Inhale deeply and begin moving one hand, then the other forward in a walking motion.
- Bring focus to your breath.
- Once your arms are fully extended in front of you, lie your forehead on the mat for 5 breath counts.
- On your next inhale, begin to walk your hands back toward your body, ending your pose in an upright seated position with your hands resting on your knees.
- Center yourself by sliding your legs out from under you and lying back.

SOMATIC YOGA FOR WEIGHT LOSS

Constructive Rest Position

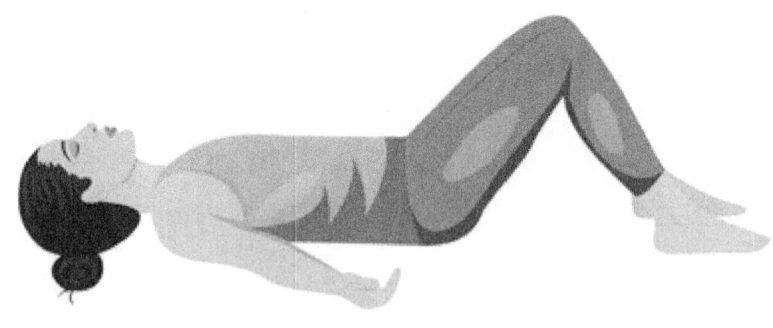

- From your supine position, bring your hands out to your side, about one hand's distance from your hips. Turn your palms so they are facing upward.
- Bend your knees and separate your feet slightly less than hip-width apart.
- Inhale deeply and begin to rock your hips from left to right in gently rolling micro-movements.
- Bring focus to your breath, repeating this movement for 10 breath counts.
- Your center is this position, pelvis flat on the mat.

Dynamic Bridge Pose

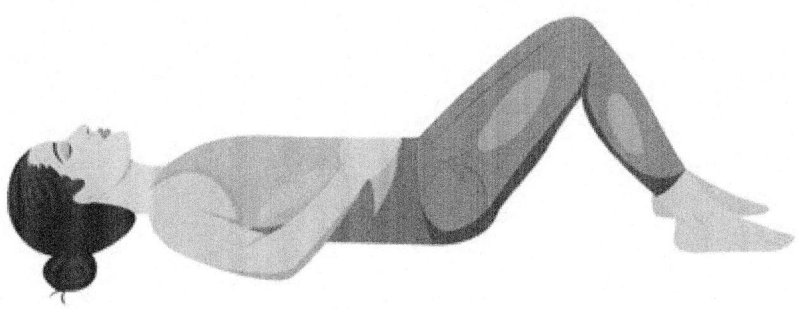

- While in your supine position, bring your hands to your pelvic area.
- Keep your knees bent and your feet rooted on the ground.
- Inhale deeply and tilt your pelvis slightly up toward your upper body in a rolling motion. This is a tiny micro-movement.
- Engage your core and hold your breath for 2 seconds in this position.
- Exhale, release your abdominal muscles, and roll your pelvis back.
- Inhale deeply again, repeating this movement 10 times.
- Return to your center by rolling over and entering the tabletop position.

Dynamic Downward Dog

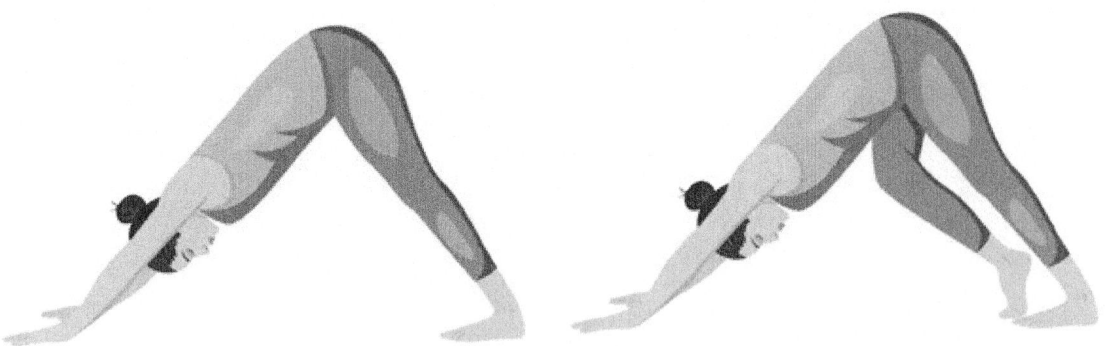

- In your tabletop position, inhale deeply and push through your feet to enter into a standard downward dog pose.
- Your body should be in an inverted "V" with your palms and feet rooted into the ground and your sit bones lifted up toward the sky.
- If you cannot straighten your legs, feel free to create more distance between your hands and your feet for greater comfort.
- Draw focus to your body, ensuring your weight is equally distributed between the hands and the feet.
- Your neck should be relaxed and the crown of the head is toward the earth. Your gaze is down and slightly forward.
- Once you are in position, inhale deeply and bend your left knee while you straighten your right leg and push your right heel down towards the floor.
- Exhale and return your left knee to a straightened position.
- Inhale once more, bending your right knee while you straighten your left leg and push your left heel down towards the floor.
- Exhale and return your right knee to a straightened position.
- Repeat this movement 10 times (5 on each side).
- Return to the center by slowly walking your hands towards your body and hinging at the hips to stand up straight.

Dynamic Tree Pose

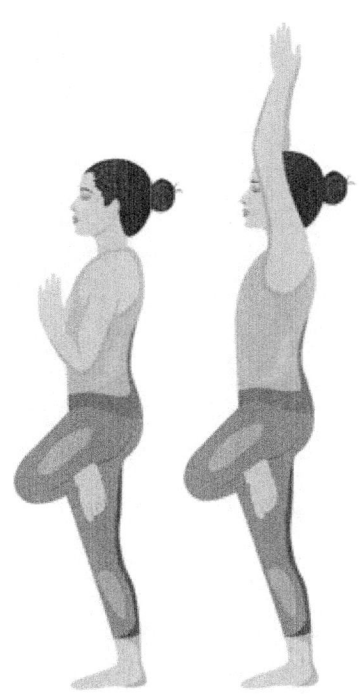

- From a standing position, shift your weight onto your right foot.
- Inhale deeply and slowly raise your right foot up your leg, resting it on your opposite ankle, calf, or thigh. Do not rest your foot on your knee.
- Exhale and as you do, bring your hands to your hands to your chest, palms together in a prayer position.
- Inhale once more and slowly lift your hands above your head, taking care to keep them in the prayer position.
- Hold your pose for 10 breath counts.
- Return to your center by slowly bringing your hands back to chest height and placing your foot back on the mat.
- Repeat your pose on the other side.
- Return to your center by placing both feet back on the mat.

SOMATIC YOGA FOR WEIGHT LOSS

Dynamic Warrior I

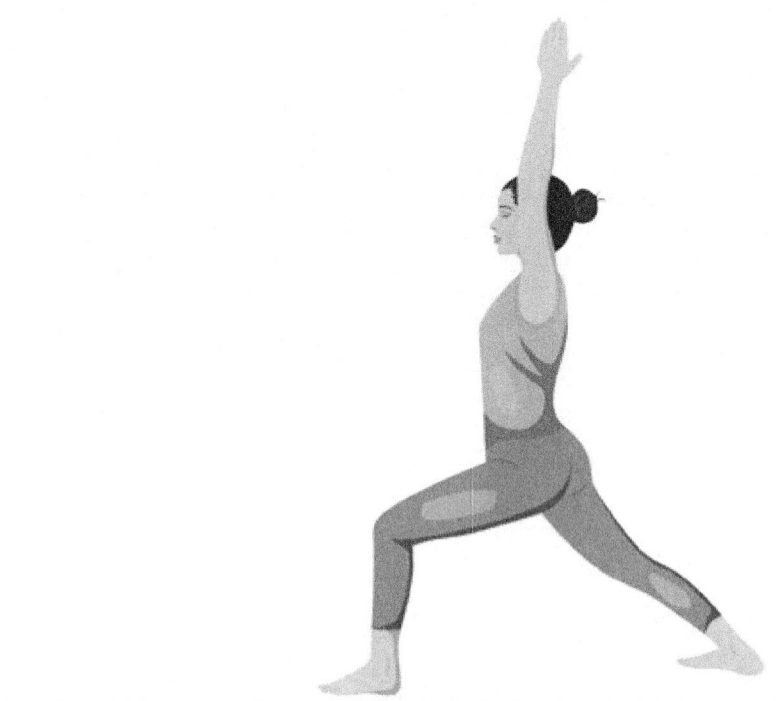

- From a standing position, your legs are in a wide stance with the feet aligned and flat on the earth.
- The back foot is at a 45-degree angle toward the front.
- Square your hips.
- Rotate your thighs toward each other.
- Bring your arms up as you inhale.
- Bend your front knee at a 90-degree angle directly above the ankle as you exhale.
- Hold this position for 5 breath counts.
- Straighten your front leg back as you inhale before bending again.
- Change your legs and repeat the movements.
- To come to your center, straighten your front leg and return to a neutral standing position.
- Bend your knees and slowly lower your body to the mat.

Gentle Fish Pose (Matsyasana)

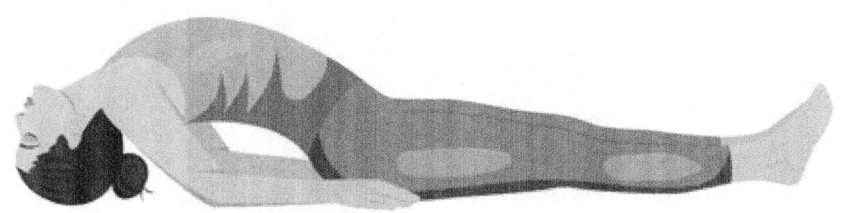

- Lie on your back, legs straight, and your arms alongside your body with your palms facing down.
- Press your shoulder blades together and slide your glutes back toward the tops of your hands.
- Once you feel safe, drop the crown of your head onto the ground and gaze behind you.
- Stay on the crown of your head and gently lift your chest toward the sky.
- Hold your pose for 10 breath counts.
- To return to your center, slide your body down flat on the mat. Place your hands at your side and bend your knees.
- Slowly return to a standing position

Gentle Standing Twists

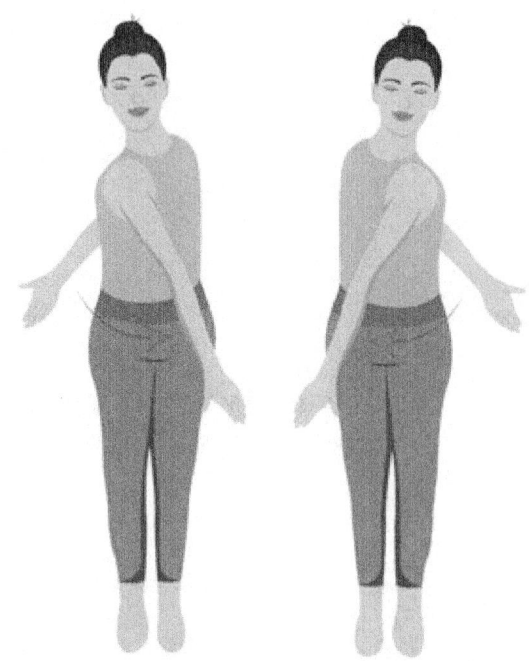

- In your standing position, bring your ankles together and place your hands at your side, palms facing your thighs.
- Inhale and gently begin to sway your upper body left and right, coordinating each swinging movement with your breath.
- Make sure your movements are controlled and that you're not twisting your spine uncomfortably.
- Complete 10 sways on each side, 20 in total.
- Return to your center by facing forward. Bend your knees and return to your mat in a seated position.

Knees to Chest Rocking

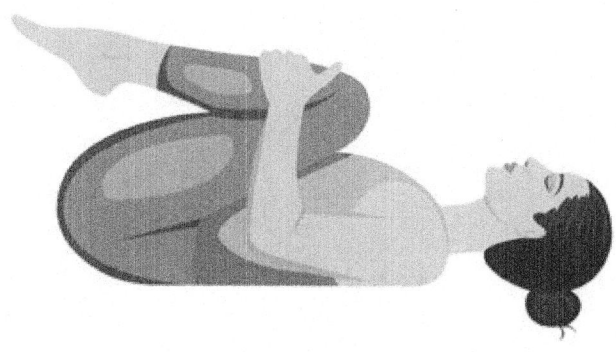

- From your seated position, lie back on your mat.
- Bring your knees against your chest, clutching them as closely as you can to your body.
- Wrap your hands around your knees securely.
- Inhale and gently begin rocking from side to side in micro-movements.
- Keep focus on your breath as you complete this movement 10 times on each side, 20 in total.
- Return to your center by placing your feet flat on the mat and bringing your hands to your side, palms on the mat in the supine position.

SOMATIC YOGA FOR WEIGHT LOSS

Leg Slides

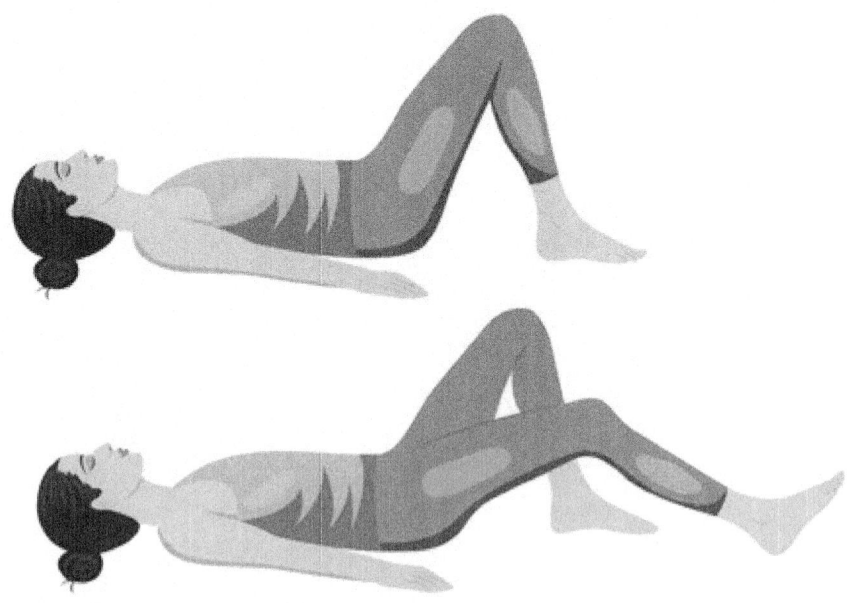

- From your supine position, bend your knees and ensure your feet are flat on the mat.
- Slide one leg out straight in front of you and flex your foot.
- Hold the position for 5 breath counts before returning your leg to the bent position.
- Slide the opposite leg out straight in front of you, flexing your foot and holding the position for 5 breath counts.
- Repeat these movements 5 times on either side, 10 in total.
- Return to your center by bringing both knees back to the bent position.

Lying Hip Release

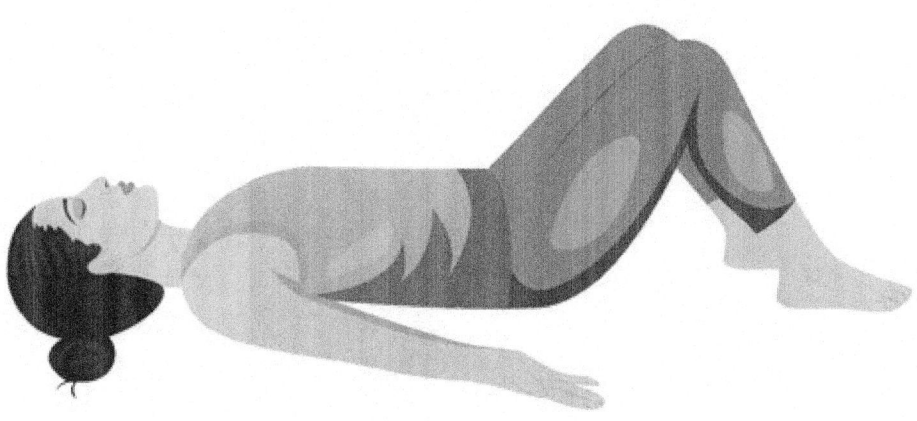

- From your supine, knees bent position, slide your arms out slightly to your sides and turn your palms so that they're facing upward.
- Inhale and separate your ankles, keeping your knees together.
- Exhale and as you do, slowly begin rocking your hips from left to right. Ensure these movements are small micro-movements.
- Continue rocking for 15 breath counts.
- Return to your center by bringing your ankles together and placing your hands on your belly.

Pelvic Clock

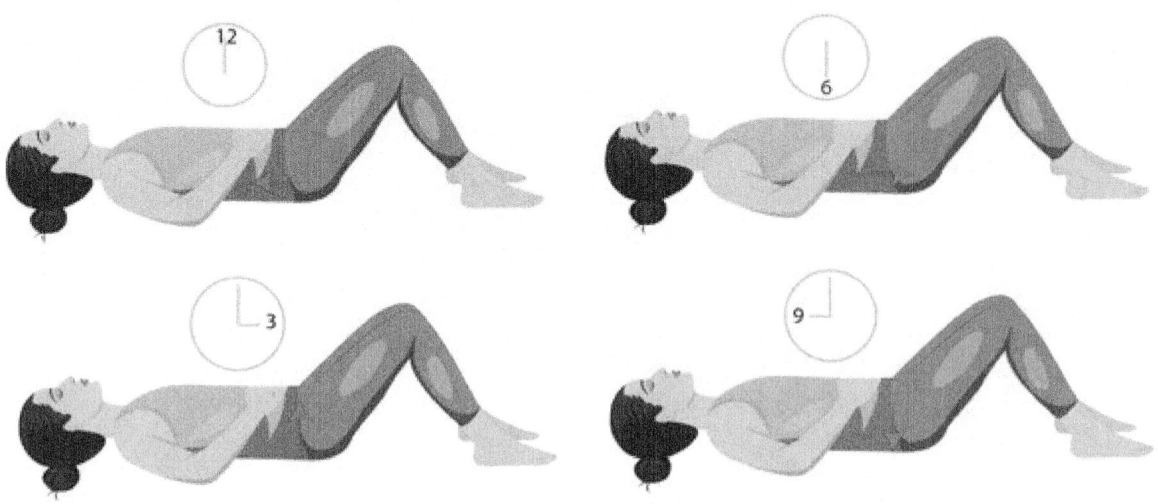

- From your supine position, hands on your belly and knees bent, begin to focus on your breath.
- As you inhale, shift your hips out to the right. Hold the position for 5 breath counts.
- On your next inhale, shift your hips down toward your feet. Hold the position for 5 breath counts.
- Inhale once more and shift your hips to the left. Hold the position for 5 breath counts.
- On your final inhale, shift your hips up to a neutral position. Hold the position for 5 breath counts.
- To return to the center, roll over onto your hands and knees into a tabletop position.

SOMATIC YOGA ROUTINES FOR STRESS MANAGEMENT, ANXIETY RELIEF, AND OVERCOMING TRAUMA

Quadruped Cat Stretch

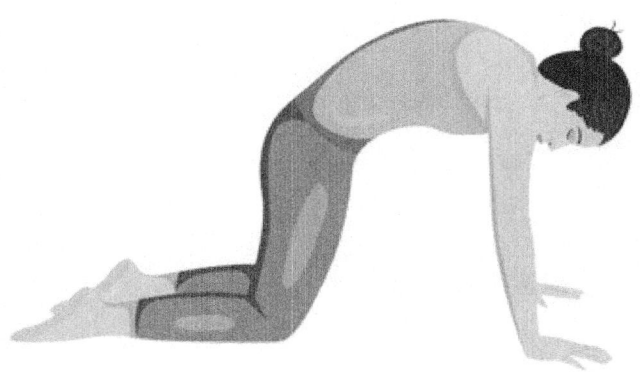

- From your tabletop position, inhale deeply while curving your lower back.
- Drop your pelvis, tilting it forward.
- Roll your shoulders forward to deepen the stretch and drop your head down toward the mat.
- Hold for 10 breath counts.
- Return to your center by returning to a tabletop position, and roll over onto your back in a supine position.

Reclined Butterfly Pose

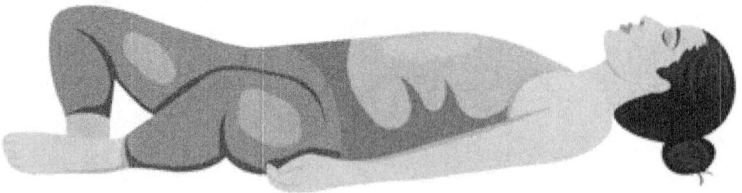

- From your supine position, bring your knees up, bending them.
- Bring your hands to your sides, resting the sides of your hands next to your sides with your palms facing up to the ceiling.
- Inhale and bring the soles of your feet together.
- Exhale and drop your knees to the side. Allow your hips to open comfortably and gaze at the ceiling.
- Engage your core, bringing focus to your breath.
- To return to your center, bring your knees together and slide your feet out straight in front of you in the supine position.

Reclined Hamstring Stretch

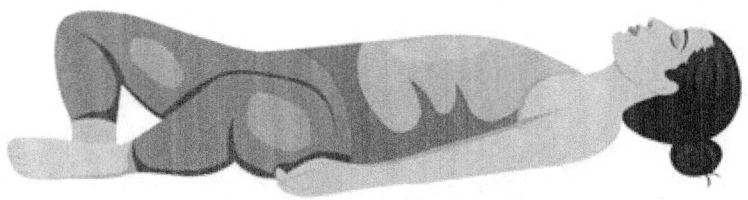

- From your supine position, inhale deeply and flex your feet.
- As you exhale, engage your core and lift your right leg up toward the ceiling.
- If you can, hold your leg in position without support. If you can't manage this, lock your hands behind your knee.
- Hold the position for 5 breath counts.
- Release your leg back to the mat and repeat the pose on the other side.
- To return to your center, bring both your legs to the mat and place your hands next to you, palms down in the supine position.

SOMATIC YOGA FOR WEIGHT LOSS

Reclined Spinal Twist

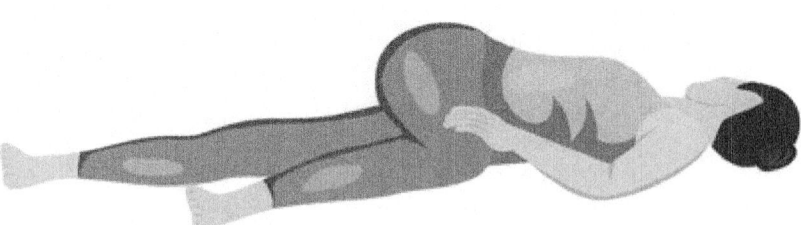

- From your supine position, bring attention to your breath.
- Inhale deeply and bend your right knee.
- As you exhale, cross your knee over your straightened leg.
- Use your left hand to put slight pressure on the bent knee to push down toward the floor.
- Keep both shoulders squared and rooted to the earth.
- Extend the opposite hand out and gaze toward that hand.
- Hold this pose for 10 breath counts.
- Return to a neutral supine position and switch sides, holding the pose for 10 breath counts.
- Come to a neutral position by returning both legs to a neutral supine position, placing your hands on the mat, and sitting up.

Seated Arm Circles

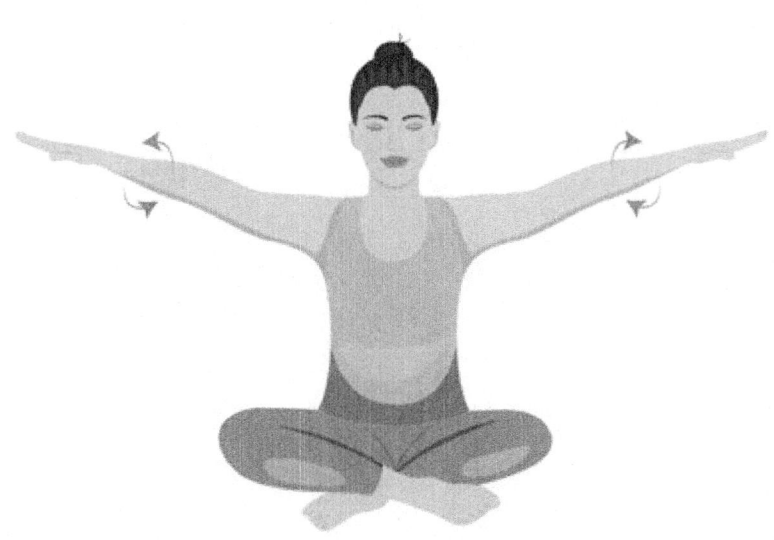

- In your seated position, cross your legs in front of you, straightening your spine.
- Inhale deeply and bring your arms out straight to your side, palms facing down toward the mat.
- Gaze forward and begin to roll your arms in a clockwise movement.
- Keep the motion small and deliberate—micro-movement.
- Complete 10 micro-movements clockwise and then anti-clockwise.
- Return to your center by dropping your arms back down to your knees.

Seated Cat-Cow

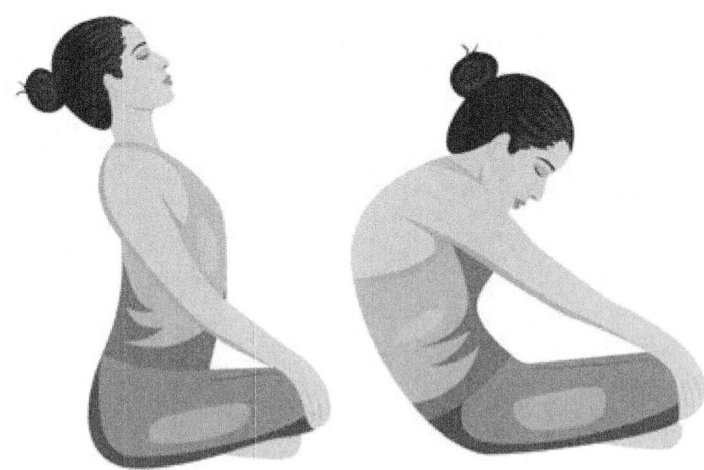

- In your seated position, inhale deeply. As you do, gently lift your head up toward the ceiling and press your chest out.
- Hold this position for 5 breath counts and release.
- Exhale deeply and as you do this, round your shoulders and drop your chin to your chest.
- Hold this position for 5 breath counts and release.
- Alternate between these two stretches 10 times.
- To return to your center, sit in a neutral position and place your hands behind you at your behind.

Seated Figure Four Stretch

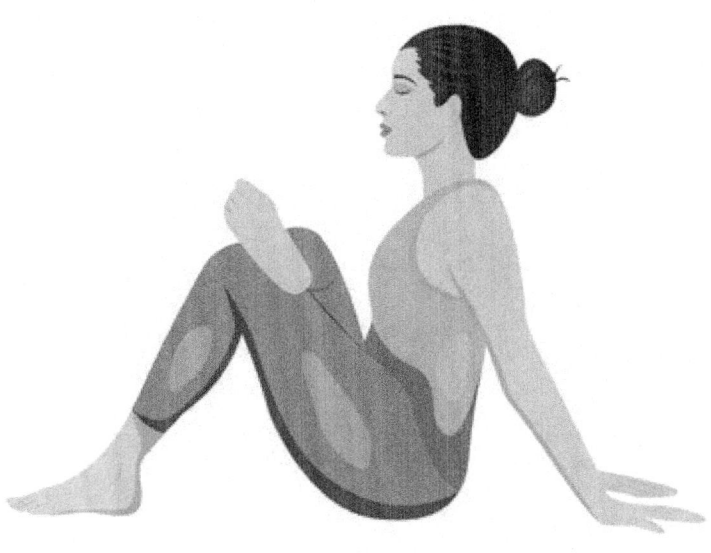

- Uncross your legs and place your feet on the mat with your knees bent.
- Lean back comfortably and inhale deeply, as you do, lift your right foot and place your foot over your left knee.
- Hold your stretch for 10 breath counts.
- Unfold your legs, returning them to the knees bent position.
- Complete the pose on the other side, holding for 10 breath counts.
- Return to your center by stretching your legs out in front of you and placing your hands on your knees.

Seated Forward Fold with Rocking

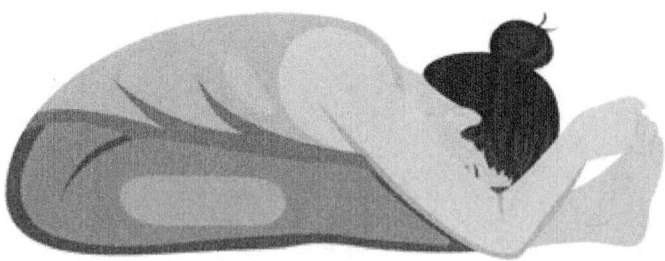

- With your legs out in front of you, flex your foot so that your toes are pointing up toward the ceiling.
- Inhale and lengthen your spine so that you're sitting up straight.
- As you exhale, slowly hinge forward from your hips, folding your body onto your thighs and your hands down toward your toes.
- If you cannot reach your toes, hold your legs, stretching where it is comfortable.
- Bring focus to your breath and hold your pose for 10 full breath cycles.
- Slowly release your pose, sitting back into an upright position.
- Place your hands at your sides on the mat and bring your legs into a crossed-legged position.

Seated Side Bend

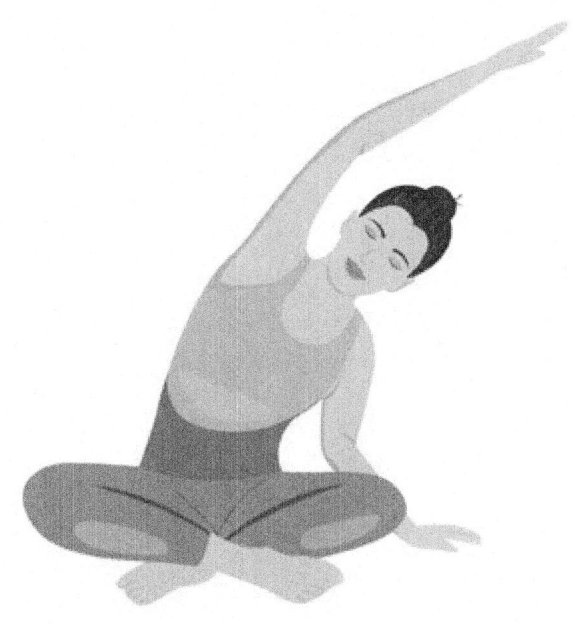

- From your cross-legged position, straighten your spine, gaze forward, and bring focus to your breath.
- Inhale deeply and as you do, bend your left elbow and raise your right arm up and over your head.
- Try to keep both palms facing the ground and your sit bones glued to the mat.
- Bend your left elbow more to deepen your stretch.
- Hold your stretch for 5 breath cycles.
- Slowly release your stretch, bringing both hands back to the mat and lengthening your spine.
- Inhale deeply and bend your right elbow, repeating the stretch on the other side for 5 breath cycles.
- Return to your center position, cross-legged.
- To set yourself up for the next pose, slide your legs out in front of you and lie back on your mat.
- Roll over onto your right side.

Side-Lying Leg Lifts

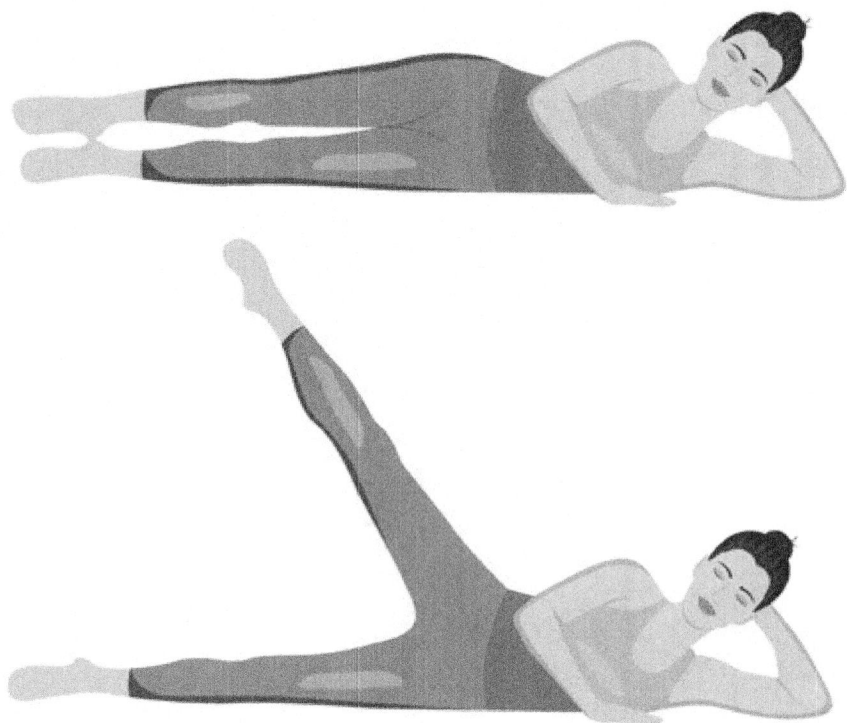

- From your right side supine position bend your right elbow, resting your head on your hand.
- Place your left hand on the mat in front of your chest.
- Make sure your legs are straight and that your knees and ankles are stacked on top of each other.
- Inhale deeply and as you do, lift your left leg up toward the ceiling.
- Hold your leg in this upward position, ensuring your knee remains straight and you're not putting pressure on your lower back.
- Bring focus to your breath and hold your leg in this position for 5 breath cycles.
- If you feel that you are strong enough, you can try to create small, pulsing, up and down movements with your lifted leg in micro-movement.
- Return your left leg to its starting position and roll over.
- Repeat the movement for 5 breath counts on the other side.
- Return to your center by rolling over onto your back in the supine position with your knees bent.

Somatic Bridge Pose

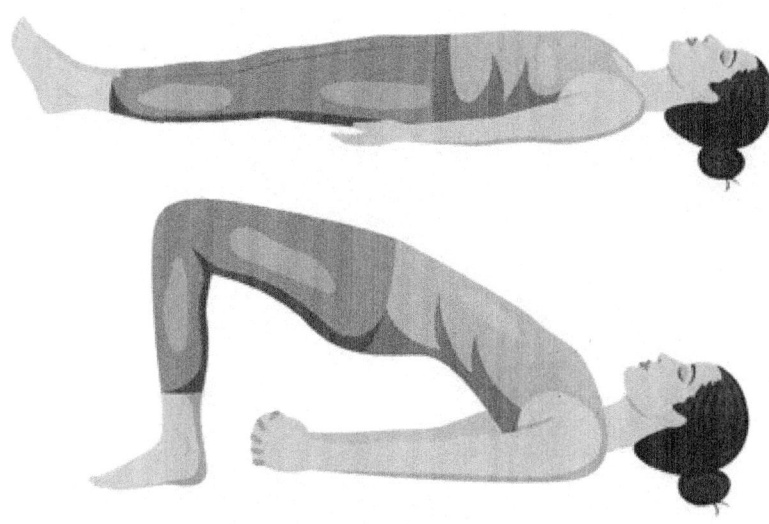

- From your legs bent supine position, bring focus to your breath.
- Inhale deeply and as you do, push up through your heels into a bridge position.
- Bring your hands under your back.
- Ensure your neck is relaxed and you are not putting strain on your back.
- Draw focus to your body and your breath and slowly start to rock back and forward, placing pressure on your shoulders then your heels, in micro-movements.
- Continue with your micro-movements for 5 full breath cycles.
- To return to your center, unclench your hands and slowly lower your body back down to the mat.

Somatic Chest Opener

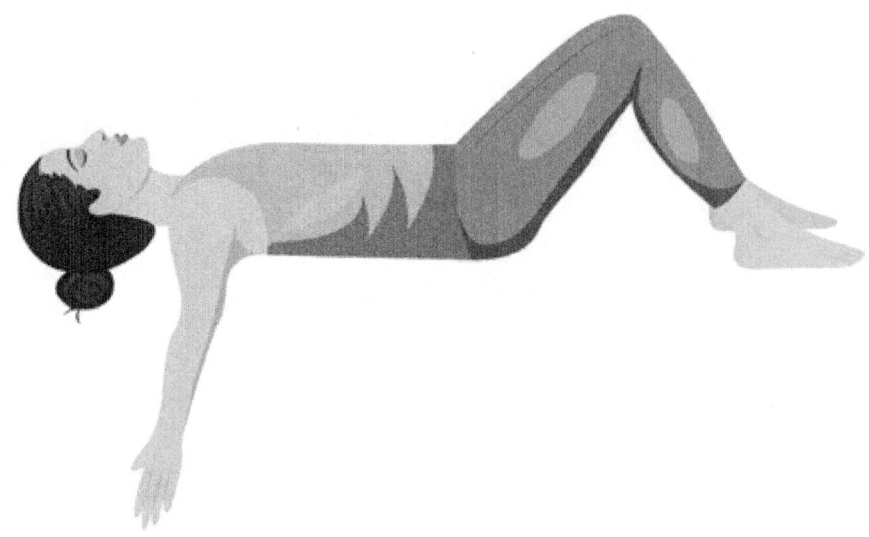

- In your knees bent supine position, slide your arms out to your sides so that your arms form a t-pose.
- Ensure your shoulders are flat on the mat and your gaze is toward the ceiling.
- Slowly inch your heels toward your glutes until your thighs are comfortably stretched.
- Inhale deeply and push your chest out toward the ceiling.
- Ensure your shoulders remain glued to the mat and that your chest-out stretch is comfortable.
- Exhale and return your chest to the mat.
- Inhale once more and push your chest out toward the ceiling.
- Continue to move between the inhale and exhale micro-movements for 10 full breath cycles.
- Return to your center by lying your shoulder and spine flat on the mat.
- Slide your legs out straight in front of you.
- Roll over onto your belly.

Somatic Cobra Pose

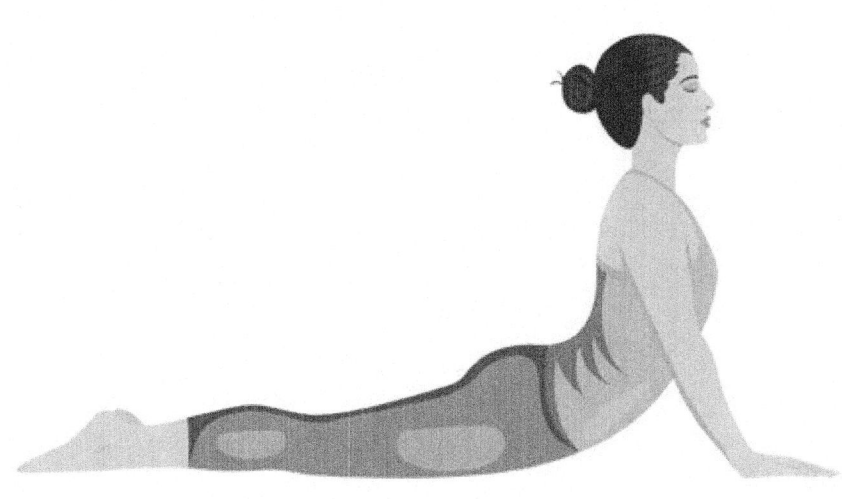

- Lie face down with your legs extended behind you, hip-width apart, and the tops of your feet resting on the mat.
- Bend your elbows and place your hands at your side, sliding them down to halfway down your rib cage.
- Hug your elbows into the sides of your body.
- Inhale and press down through the hands and lift your head and chest off the floor.
- Draw your shoulders back and your heart forward keeping your head in a natural position gazing straight forward.
- Roll your shoulders back and away from your ears as you begin to straighten your arms to a position that is comfortable for your spine.
- Hold your position for 10 full breath cycles.
- To release your pose, bend your elbows and gently lower your upper body to the mat.
- Return your arms to a neutral position and roll over onto your back.
- Inhale deeply and sit up before bending your knees and standing up.

SOMATIC YOGA FOR WEIGHT LOSS

Somatic Crescent Lunge

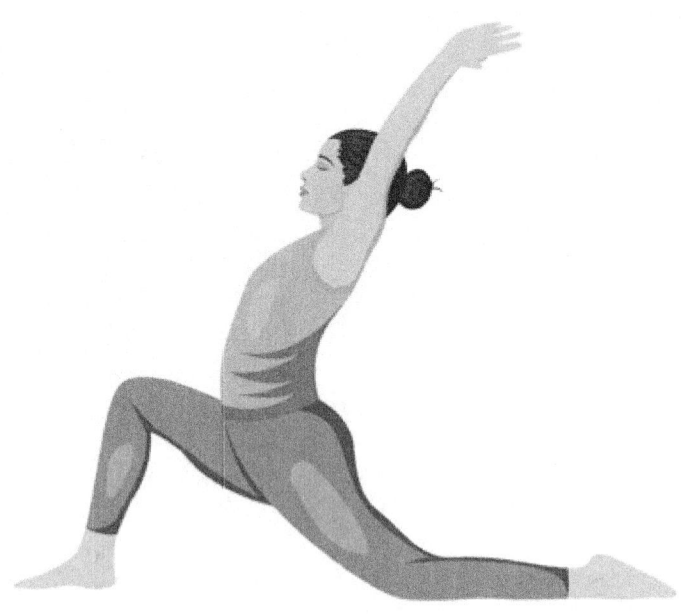

- Move to the top of your mat and stand in a neutral position with your hands at your sides.
- Take a large step forward with your right leg, planting your feet flat on the mat. Ensure both feet are facing forward.
- Place your front foot flat on the floor, and your front knee stacked directly over your heel.
- Inhale and slowly bend your front knee, keeping your back leg as straight as possible.
- Gradually lower your back leg, flattening the top of your left foot on the mat until your right knee is stacked over your right ankle.
- Inhale deeply and sweep your hands up toward the ceiling, palms facing each other.
- Hold your position for 5 full breath counts before dropping your hands back down to your sides and standing up.
- Take a large step forward with your left leg now, and ensure both your feet are planted firmly on the mat.
- Repeat your pose on the left side for 5 full breath counts before dropping your hands back down to your sides and standing up.
- Return to your center by standing in a neutral position.

SOMATIC YOGA ROUTINES FOR STRESS MANAGEMENT, ANXIETY RELIEF, AND OVERCOMING TRAUMA

Somatic Forward Fold

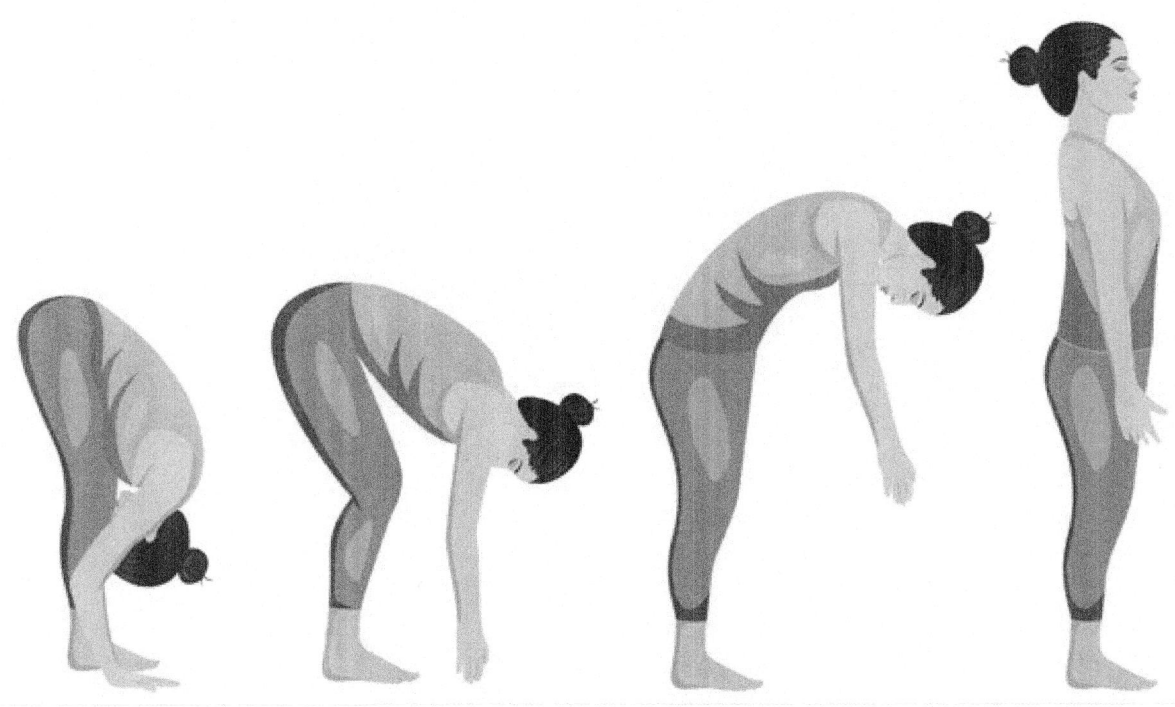

- From your neutral standing position, stand upright with your feet slightly less than hip-width apart, arms at your sides.
- Inhale and bend forward, hinging at your hips.
- Try to keep your back straight and let your arms hang down towards the mat.
- Draw focus to your breath, and hold your forward bend for 5 full breath cycles.
- On your sixth inhale, bend your knees slightly, bringing your hands to the mat.
- Exhale and straighten your arms as you slowly begin to roll up, vertebra by vertebra, starting from your lower back.
- Continue rolling up through your mid-back and upper back.
- Finally, lift your head and return to an upright standing position.
- Return to your center by opening your legs hip-width apart. Drop to your knees and enter into a tabletop position.

SOMATIC YOGA FOR WEIGHT LOSS

Somatic Frog Pose

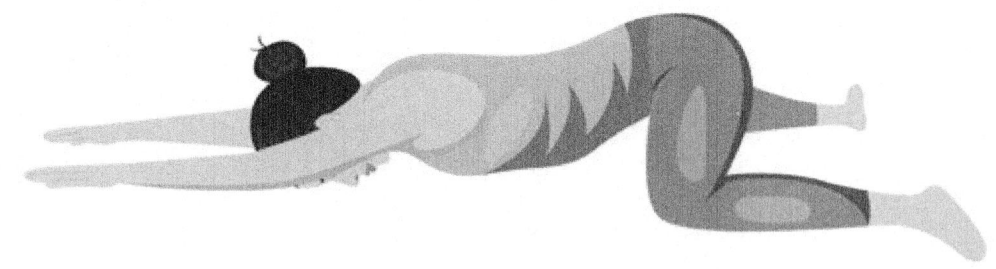

- From your tabletop position, inhale deeply and as you exhale, slowly start walking your arms forward on the mat, palms facing down.
- Slowly begin spreading your knees apart wider than hip-width, turning your feet out.
- Draw focus to your breath and allow your hips to sink back toward your heels.
- Relax your lower back, letting it curve naturally.
- Hold your pose for 5 full breath cycles, allowing your body to settle deeper with each exhale.
- To release, slowly bring your knees together and sit back on your heels before returning to a neutral position.
- Slide your legs out from under you and lie flat on your belly.

Somatic Half-Bow Pose

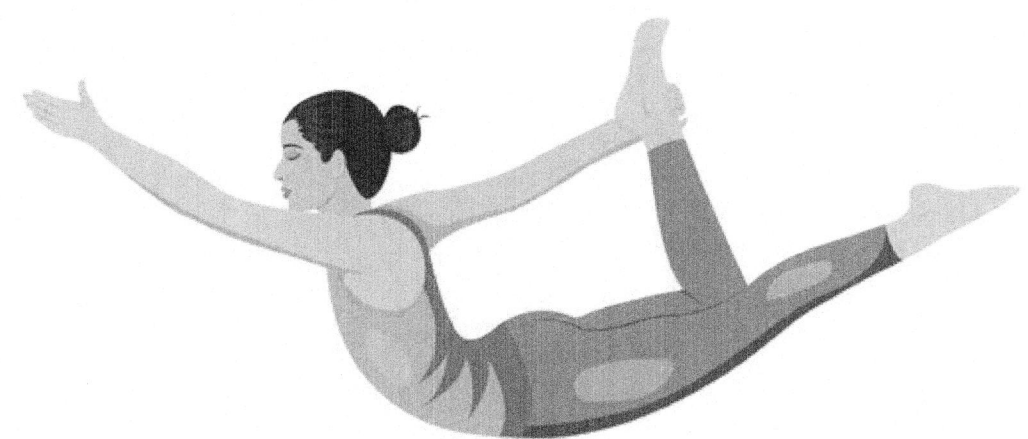

- From your position lying face down, bend your knees, bringing your heels towards your buttocks.
- Reach your arms back and grasp the outside of your right foot with your right arm. If this is too difficult to do, feel free to use a strap, blanket, or towel to extend your reach.
- Inhale deeply, and as you exhale, lift your chest, thighs, and feet off the mat simultaneously.
- Draw focus to your breath and engage your back muscles to lift your chest higher.
- Press your foot into your hand to create a deep backbend, opening your chest and shoulders.
- If you can, lift your left arm out straight in front of you.
- Hold your pose for 5 full breath cycles, allowing your body to find stability and depth with each exhale.
- Keep your gaze forward or slightly upward, maintaining length in the back of your neck.
- To release, slowly lower your chest, thighs, and foot back to the mat on an exhale.
- Repeat your pose on the left side for 5 full breath cycles.
- Return to your center and then push up into a tabletop position.
- Kneel back and stand up.

SOMATIC YOGA FOR WEIGHT LOSS

Somatic Hip Rolls

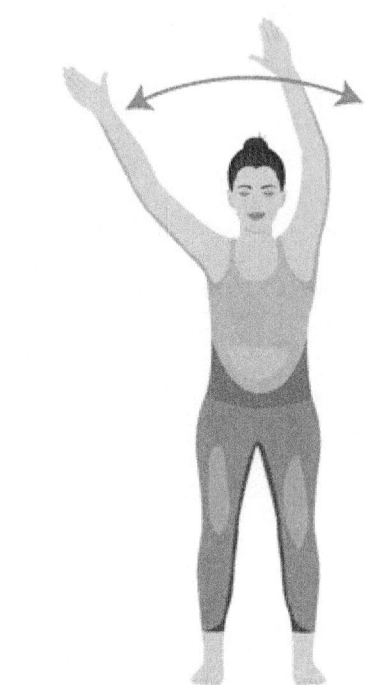

- From your neutral standing position, stand upright with your feet hip-width apart, arms at your sides.
- Inhale deeply and raise your arms overhead, palms facing each other.
- As you exhale, bend your knees slightly and begin to sway your hips to the right while reaching your arms to the left.
- Inhale as you return to the center, keeping your arms overhead.
- On your next exhale, sway your hips to the left while reaching your arms to the right.
- Draw focus to your breath, coordinating each sway with your exhale and each return to center with your inhale.
- Continue this fluid movement for 10 full breath cycles, allowing your body to loosen and relax with each sway.
- Keep your feet grounded and knees slightly bent throughout the movement.
- To finish, return to your neutral standing center on an inhale, then slowly lower your arms to your sides on an exhale.

Standing Pelvic Tilts

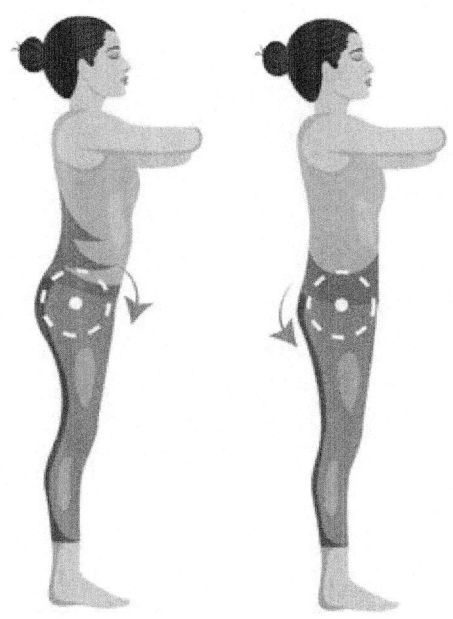

- From your neutral standing position, stand with your feet hip-width apart, and knees slightly bent.
- Bring your arms up to your chest, crossing them lightly.
- Inhale deeply, and as you exhale, tilt your pelvis backward (posterior tilt), tucking your tailbone under.
- As you do this, feel your lower back flattening and your abdominal muscles engaging.
- On your next inhale, tilt your pelvis forward (anterior tilt), arching your lower back slightly.
- Draw focus to your breath, coordinating each tilt with your breath cycle.
- Continue this gentle rocking motion for 10 full breath cycles, moving smoothly between posterior and anterior tilts.
- Keep your upper body relatively still, focusing the movement in your pelvis and lower back.
- Maintain a soft bend in your knees throughout the exercise.
- To finish, return to a neutral pelvic position on an exhale.
- Set yourself up for your next pose by bending your knees and lowering yourself to the mat in a kneeling position.

Somatic Pigeon Pose

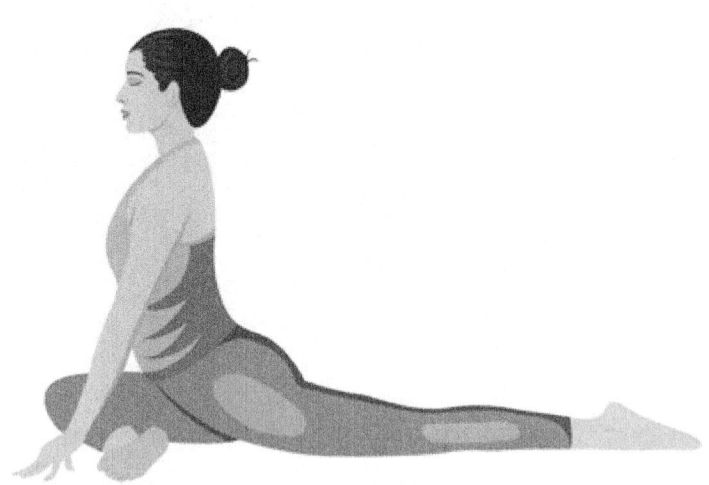

- From your kneeling position, inhale deeply and bring your right knee forward towards your right wrist.
- Keep your hands flat on the mat on either side of your right knee.
- As you exhale, slide your right foot towards your left hip, angling it as comfortable.
- Extend your left leg straight back behind you, the top of the foot resting on the mat.
- Inhale and lengthen your spine, lifting through the crown of your head.
- Draw focus to your breath, allowing your hips to sink deeper with each exhale.
- Keep your hips square to the front of the mat as much as possible.
- Hold this pose for 5 full breath cycles, relaxing deeper into the stretch with each breath.
- To release, slide your right leg back and bring your left leg in so that you return to kneeling.
- Repeat on the other side, bringing your left knee forward and extending your right leg back.
- Hold for 5 full breath cycles before returning to your center.
- Lean forward and place both hands on the mat before lifting your glutes and entering into a tabletop position.

Somatic Plank Pose

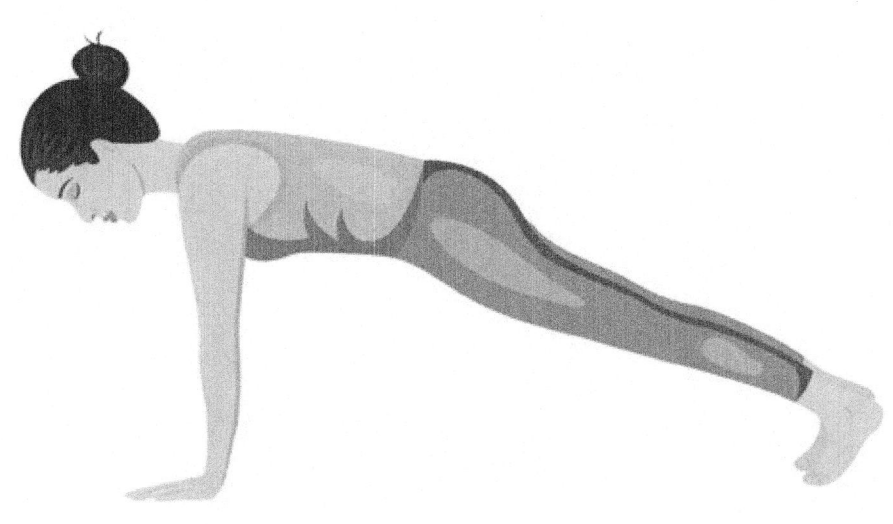

- From your tabletop position, inhale deeply and engage your core muscles.
- As you exhale, step your feet back one at a time, extending your legs fully.
- Align your body in a straight line from your heels to the crown of your head.
- Draw focus to your breath, maintaining a steady and even breathing pattern and ensuring your core is engaged.
- Keep your palms flat on the mat, directly under your shoulders, fingers spread wide.
- Engage your thighs, drawing your navel towards your spine for further core stability.
- Hold this pose for 15 full breath cycles, maintaining a strong and steady posture.
- Keep your gaze fixed on a point between your hands, maintaining a neutral neck position.
- With each inhale, imagine lengthening your spine; with each exhale, reinforce your core engagement.
- To release, slowly lower your knees back to the mat, returning to the tabletop position on an exhale.
- Slide your legs out in front of you to enter into a seated position.
- Place your hands on the mat behind you and lie down in a supine position with your arms resting at your sides.

Somatic Scapula Mobilization

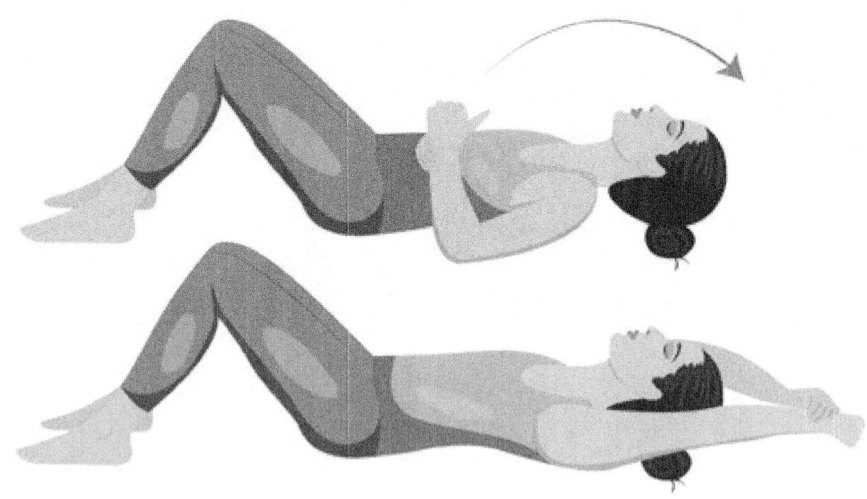

- From your supine position (lying on your back), bend your knees and place your feet flat on the mat.
- Inhale deeply and bend your elbows.
- Hold your right wrist with your left hand.
- On your next inhale extend your arms straight up towards the ceiling, ensuring your right wrist is still firmly grasped.
- As you exhale, lower your arms overhead, keeping your right arm straight, until they rest on the floor above your head.
- Draw focus to your breath and the movement of your shoulder blades.
- Hold your stretch for 5 full breath cycles.
- Keep your lower back pressed into the mat throughout the exercise.
- Maintain the bend in your knees, feet flat on the floor, to support your lower back.
- To finish, bring your arms back to your sides on an inhale, and relax completely on your exhale.
- Repeat your exercise on the other side, clasping your left wrist with your right hand.
- Return to your center by pushing up through your hands and entering into a seated position.
- Bend your legs and enter into a cross-legged seat.

Somatic Seated Twist

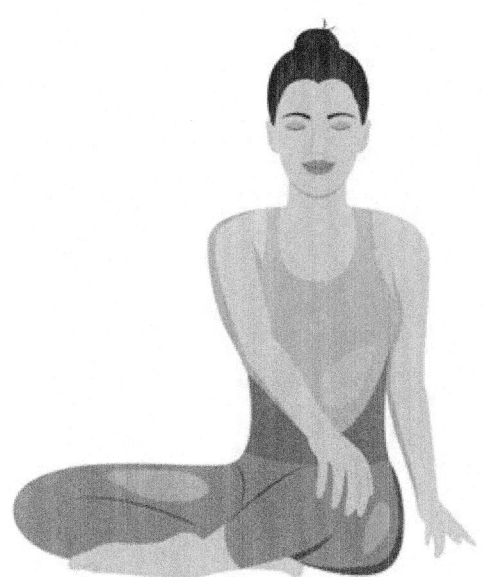

- From your cross-legged seated position, inhale deeply and lengthen your spine, sitting tall.
- As you exhale, place your right hand on the floor behind you, close to your hips.
- Inhale again, and as you exhale, bring your left hand to the outside of your right knee.
- Draw focus to your breath, using each inhale to lengthen your spine.
- On each exhale, gently deepen the twist, rotating from your core.
- Keep your sit bones grounded and your spine long throughout the twist.
- Turn your head to look over your right shoulder, if comfortable for your neck.
- Hold this twist for 5 full breath cycles, allowing your body to relax deeper into the pose with each exhale.
- To release, slowly unwind on an inhale, returning to the center.
- Repeat on the other side, placing your left hand behind you and your right hand to the outer left knee.
- Bring your legs out in front of you, knees bent, and push up through your hands and quads into a standing position.

SOMATIC YOGA FOR WEIGHT LOSS

Somatic Side Stretch

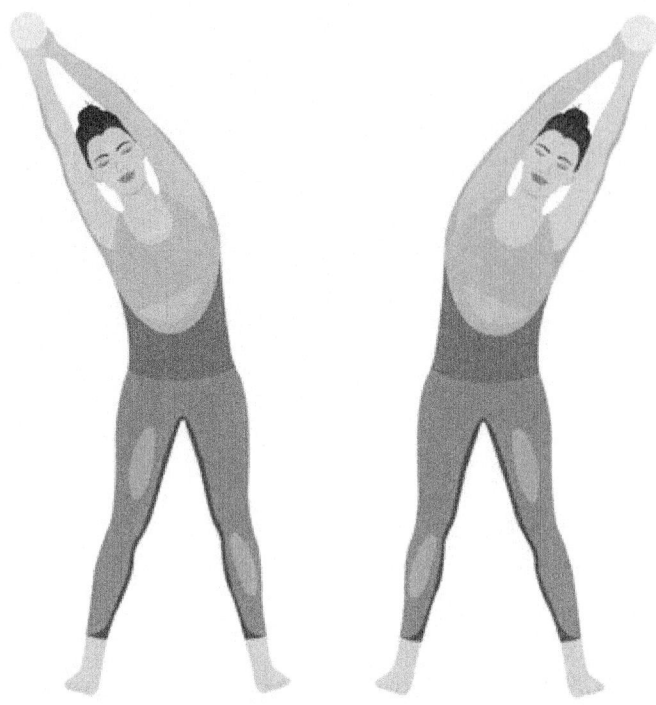

- From your neutral standing position, take a small step out so that you're standing with feet hip-width apart, and arms at your sides.
- Inhale deeply and raise both arms overhead, palms facing each other.
- As you exhale, interlace your fingers and extend your arms fully, pointing your index fingers up.
- Draw focus to your breath and engage your core for stability.
- On your next inhale, lengthen your spine and reach up through your fingertips.
- As you exhale, begin to bend to your right side, creating a long curve with the left side of your body.
- Hold this position for a full breath cycle, then begin to bend toward your toes and release in micro-movement for 5 full breath cycles.
- On your sixth inhale, slightly straighten your torso.
- Repeat your exercise on the left side.
- To finish, release your arms down to your sides on an exhale, returning to the starting position.
- Bend your knees and come back to the mat in a seated position with your knees bent in front of you.
- Place your hands on the mat behind you and lower your body to the mat in a knees bent supine position.

Somatic Shoulder Bridge

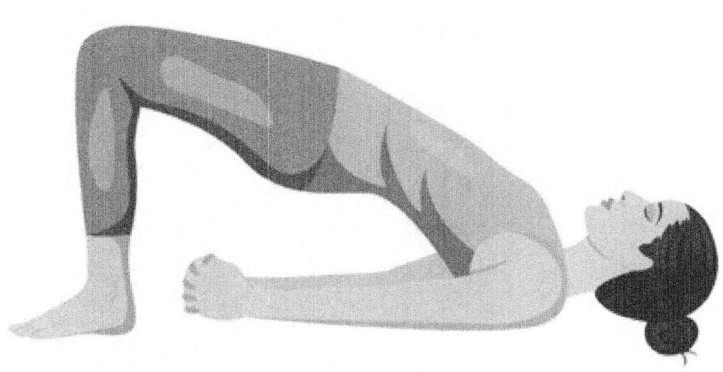

- From your supine position, bend your knees and place your feet flat on the mat, hip-width apart.
- Extend your arms along your sides, palms facing down.
- Inhale deeply, and as you exhale, engage your core and press your lower back into the mat entering into a traditional bridge pose.
- On your next inhale, slowly peel your spine off the mat, starting with your tailbone.
- Continue to roll up vertebrae by vertebrae until you're resting on your shoulder blades.
- Draw focus to your breath and the engagement of your glutes and hamstrings.
- Lift your hips high, creating a straight line from your knees to your shoulders.
- Unlike a regular bridge, keep your upper back and shoulders firmly on the mat.
- Hold this position for 5 full breath cycles, maintaining the elevation of your hips.
- To add intensity, you can rise onto your toes, lifting your heels off the mat.
- To release, slowly lower your spine back to the mat on an exhale, vertebra by vertebra.
- Finish by relaxing completely, allowing your lower back to soften into the mat.
- To return to your center, push through your hands and hinge at your hips to enter into a seated position with your knees bent.

SOMATIC YOGA FOR WEIGHT LOSS

Somatic Shoulder Shrugs

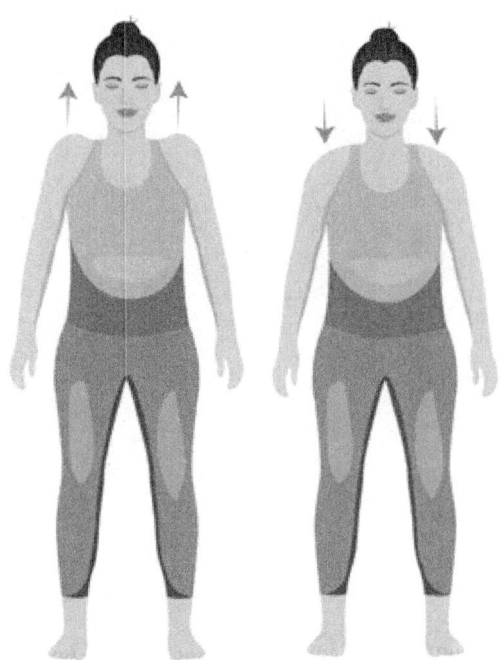

- From your seated position with your knees bent, sit tall with your spine elongated.
- Place your hands on your thighs or let them rest by your sides.
- Inhale deeply and as you exhale, drop your shoulders away from your ears.
- Draw focus to your breath and the sensation in your shoulder muscles.
- On your next inhale, slowly lift your shoulders up towards your ears.
- As you exhale, gently lower your shoulders back down.
- Continue this shrugging motion for 10 full breath cycles, coordinating the movement with your breath.
- Keep your neck relaxed and your gaze forward throughout the exercise.
- For added benefit, hold the shrug at the top for a moment before releasing.
- On your final exhale, let your shoulders settle into a relaxed, neutral position.
- Take a moment to notice any changes in tension or sensation in your neck and shoulder area.
- Lean forward and place your hands on the mat in front of you. Hinge at the hips and enter into a tabletop position.

Somatic Sunbird Pose

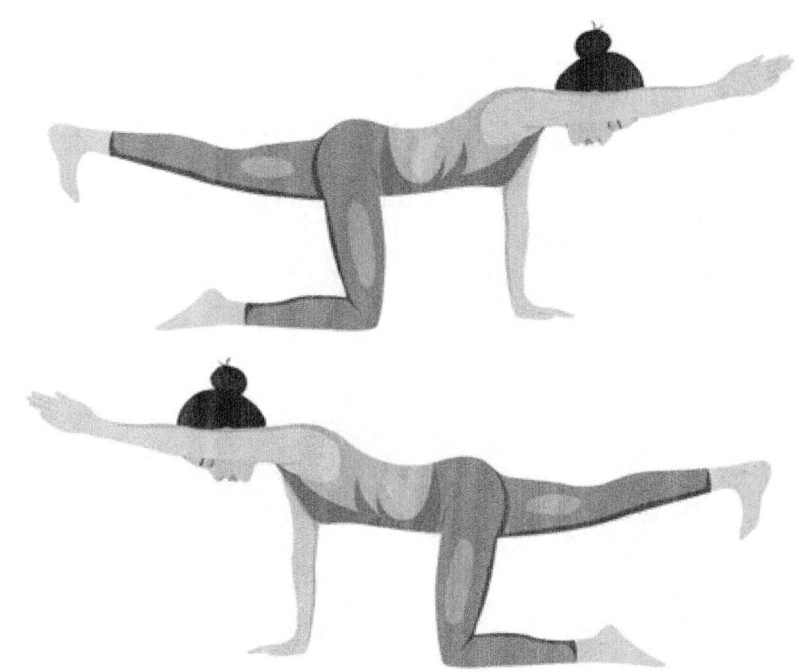

- From your tabletop position, ensure your wrists are under your shoulders and knees under your hips.
- Inhale deeply, and as you exhale, engage your core muscles.
- On your next inhale, slowly extend your right arm forward and your left leg back.
- Draw focus to your breath and maintain balance through your core.
- Aim to bring your right arm and left leg parallel to the floor.
- Keep your hips level and square to the mat, avoiding any rotation.
- Hold this position for 5 full breath cycles, maintaining a strong and steady posture.
- Keep your gaze down between your supporting hand and knee for neck alignment.
- With each inhale, imagine lengthening through your fingertips and heel.
- To release, slowly lower your arm and leg back to the starting position on an exhale.
- Repeat on the other side, extending your left arm and right leg.
- Lower your body to the mat and roll over onto your back with your knees bent.

Somatic Twists

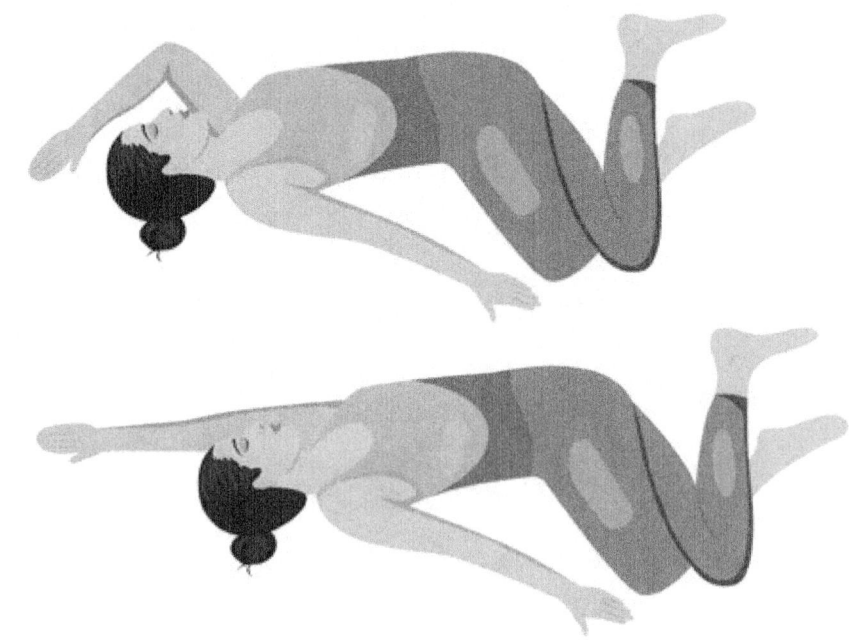

- From your supine position, bent knee position, cross your right leg over your left.
- Extend your right arm up overhead and allow your left arm to remain at your side, about half an arm's length from your torso.
- Inhale deeply, and as you exhale, drop both knees to the left side of your body.
- Keep both shoulders pressed firmly into the mat as you twist.
- Draw focus to your breath, allowing the twist to deepen with each exhale.
- Turn your head to the right if it is comfortable for your neck.
- Hold this twist for 5 full breath cycles, feeling the stretch along your spine and obliques.
- On your next inhale, slowly bring your knees back to the center.
- Exhale and then cross your left leg over your right, bring your left arm up overhead, and reposition your right arm about half an arm's width from your torso.
- Drop both knees to the right side, turning your head to the right if comfortable.
- Hold for another 5 breath cycles on this side.
- To finish, inhale as you bring your knees back to center, untwist your legs, and exhale as you roll over into a tabletop position.

SOMATIC YOGA ROUTINES FOR STRESS MANAGEMENT, ANXIETY RELIEF, AND OVERCOMING TRAUMA

Somatic Tabletop Cat-Cow

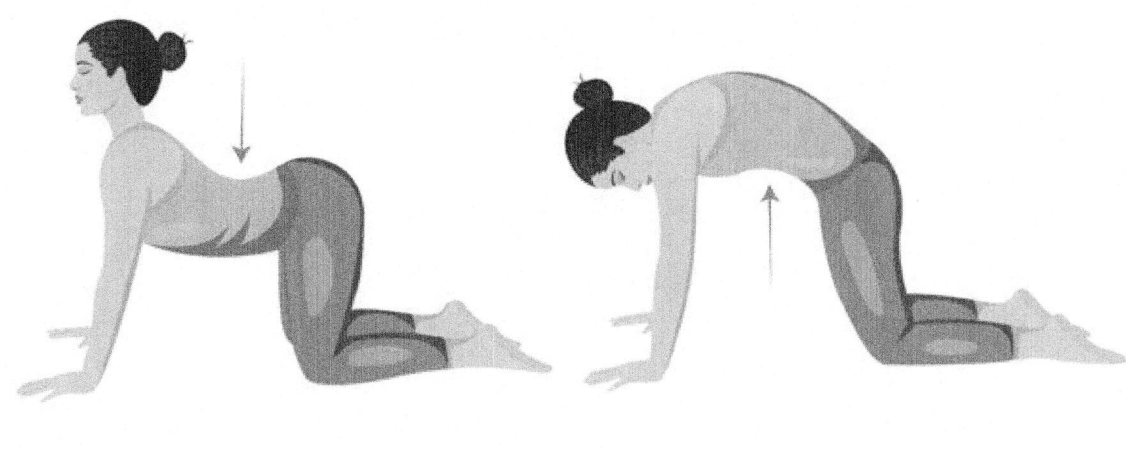

- From your tabletop position, ensure your wrists are under your shoulders and knees under your hips.
- Inhale deeply, and as you exhale, move into Cow pose with your spine dropped toward the mat and your chest and tailbone towards the ceiling.
- Draw focus to your body and begin to rock your body forward and backward, shifting your weight slightly onto and off of your hands.
- Rock for 3 full breath cycles and draw focus to your breath and the fluidity of the movement.
- On your next inhale, transition to the cat pose, rounding your spine towards the ceiling, and tucking your chin to your chest.
- As you round, rock your body forward and backward, shifting your weight onto and off of your knees.
- Continue this rocking for 3 full breath cycles.
- Inhale and transition to cow pose once more, repeating cat and cow two more times (3 cycles).
- Once you're done, sit back onto your knees and push up using your hands and thighs to enter into a standing position.

Somatic Warrior II

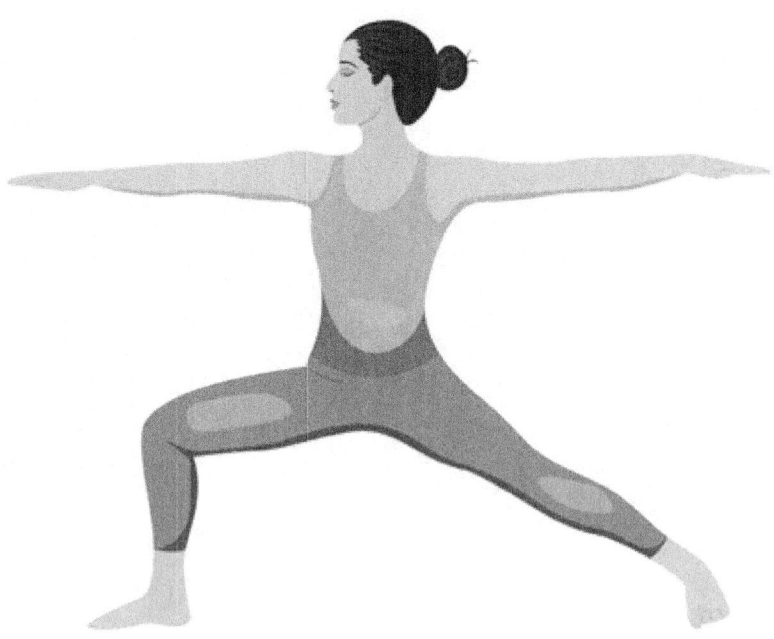

- From your neutral standing position, step your feet wide apart, about 3-4 feet.
- Inhale deeply, and as you exhale, turn your right foot out 90 degrees and your left foot in slightly.
- On your next inhale, raise your arms parallel to the floor, palms facing down.
- As you exhale, bend your right knee over your right ankle, and thigh parallel to the floor if possible.
- Draw focus to your breath and the strength in your legs.
- Gaze over your right fingertips, keeping your shoulders relaxed away from your ears.
- Sink your hips low, keeping your torso upright and core engaged.
- Press the outer edge of your back foot firmly into the mat for stability.
- Hold this pose for 5 full breath cycles, maintaining a strong and steady posture.
- With each inhale, lengthen your spine; with each exhale, sink deeper into the pose.
- To release, inhale as you straighten your right leg and lower your arms.
- Exhale and turn to face forward, then repeat on the left side.
- To return to your center, bend your knees and drop to the mat. Slide your feet out in front of you and lie down in the supine position.

SOMATIC YOGA ROUTINES FOR STRESS MANAGEMENT, ANXIETY RELIEF, AND OVERCOMING TRAUMA

Somatic Wave

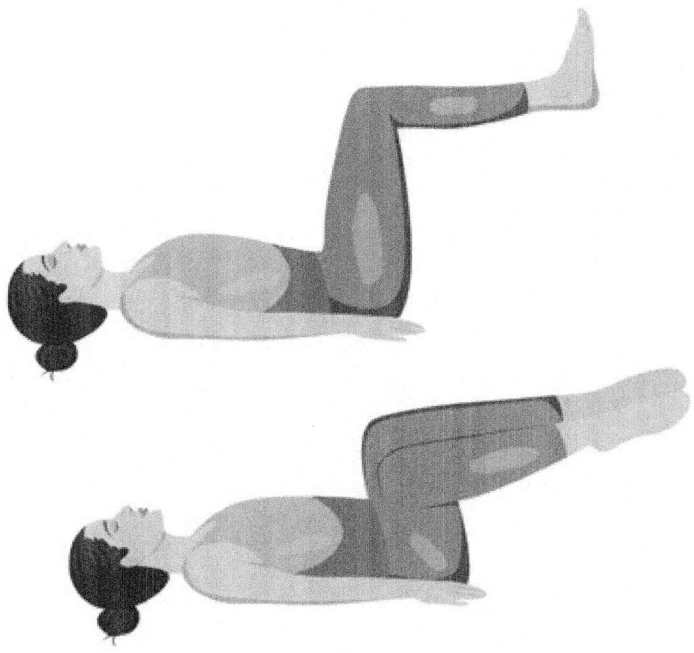

- From your supine position (lying on your back), bend your knees and lift your feet from the mat, bending at the pelvis.
- Place your arms at your sides, palms down on the mat.
- Inhale deeply, and as you exhale, draw focus to your breath and the engagement of your core muscles.
- On your next inhale, begin to rock your hips from side to side ensuring that your spine remains on the mat and that only your glutes are being lifted.
- Keep your movements small and controlled.
- Continue this rocking motion for 15 full breath cycles, coordinating each movement with your breath.
- To return to your center, lower your legs to the mat and straighten them out in front of you. Roll over onto your belly.

Sphinx Pose

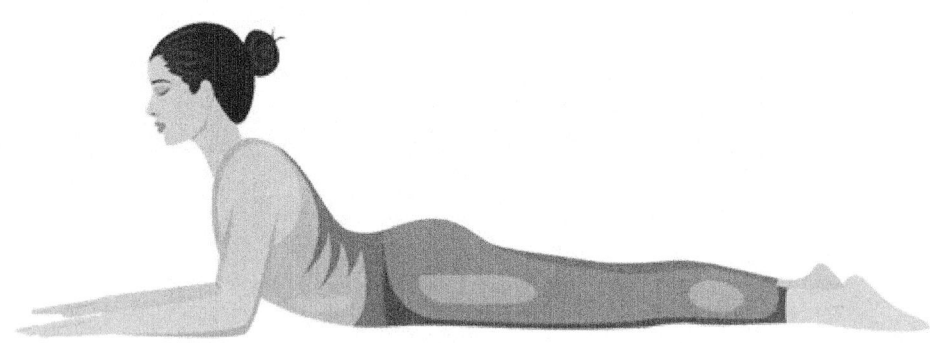

- From your prone position (lying on your stomach), extend your legs straight behind you.
- Place your forearms on the mat, elbows directly under your shoulders.
- Inhale deeply, and as you exhale, press your forearms into the mat to lift your upper body.
- Draw focus to your breath and the gentle arch in your lower back.
- Keep your legs engaged, pressing the tops of your feet into the mat.
- Lengthen through your spine, drawing your chest forward and up.
- Relax your shoulders away from your ears, keeping your neck long.
- Hold this pose for 15 full breath cycles, maintaining a steady and comfortable position.
- With each inhale, imagine lengthening your spine; with each exhale, settle deeper into the pose.
- Keep your gaze soft and directed slightly downward to maintain proper neck alignment.
- To release, slowly lower your upper body back to the mat on an exhale.
- Rest your forehead on the mat and relax your arms by your sides.
- Return to your center by sliding your knees under you to enter into a tabletop position.
- Sit back on your heels and stand up.

Standing Forward Bend with Swaying

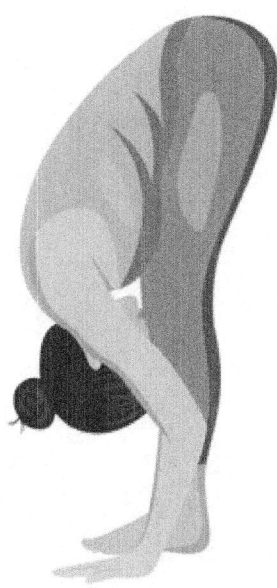

- From your neutral standing position, stand with your feet hip-width apart, arms at your sides.
- Inhale deeply, and as you exhale, hinge at your hips to fold forward.
- Allow your upper body to hang heavy, bending your knees slightly if needed.
- Let your arms and head dangle towards the floor, releasing tension in your neck and shoulders.
- Draw focus to your breath and the stretch along the back of your legs.
- Begin a gentle swaying motion—as you inhale, sway your upper body slightly to the right, and as you exhale, sway to the left.
- Continue this swaying motion for 15 full breath cycles, moving slowly and mindfully.
- Allow the sway to increase the stretch on alternating sides of your back and legs.
- Keep your core gently engaged to protect your lower back.
- Gradually decrease the sway, coming back to the center.
- To release, slowly roll up to standing, vertebra by vertebra, on an inhale.
- Let your head be the last to come up, returning to your starting position.
- To return to your center, bend your knees and come to the mat. Slide your legs out in front of you and lie down.

SOMATIC YOGA FOR WEIGHT LOSS

Supine Arm Circles

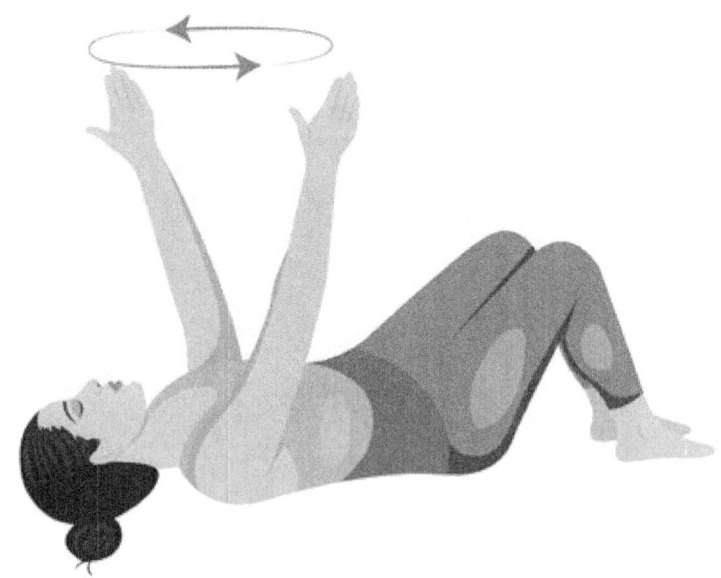

- From your supine position (lying on your back), bend your knees and place your feet flat on the mat.
- Inhale deeply, and as you exhale, press your lower back into the mat.
- Extend your arms straight up towards the ceiling, palms facing each other.
- Draw focus to your breath and the stability of your core and shoulder blades.
- Begin small circular movements with your arms—as you inhale, circle your arms clockwise, and as you exhale, reverse the direction to counter-clockwise.
- Gradually increase the size of the circles, maintaining control and keeping your shoulder blades pressed into the mat.
- Continue this circular motion for 15 full breath cycles in each direction.
- Keep your core engaged throughout the exercise to support your lower back.
- If comfortable, you can progress to larger circles, allowing your arms to brush the floor at the bottom of the movement.
- To finish, slowly bring your arms back to the starting position on an exhale.
- Relax your arms by your sides, taking a moment to notice any sensations in your shoulders.

Supine PSOAS Release

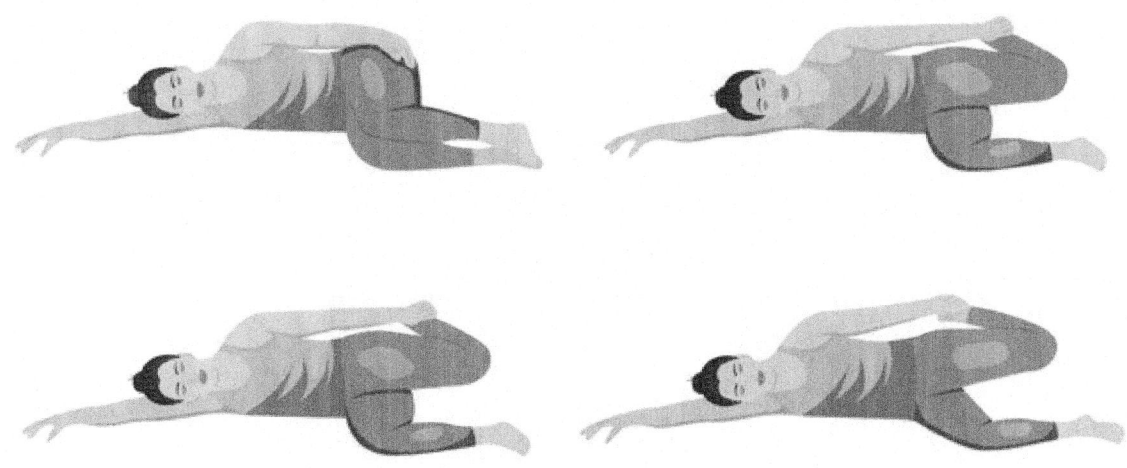

- From your supine position (lying on your back), bend both knees and place your feet flat on the mat.
- Inhale deeply, and as you exhale, drop both knees to the right side of your body, allowing your shoulders to follow.
- Draw focus to your breath and the sensation in your left hip and lower back.
- Extend your right arm out underneath you and rest your head on your arm.
- On your next inhale, reach your left arm back as you deepen the bend in your left leg.
- If you can, hold your left foot or ankle.
- Hold this stretch for 5 full breath cycles.
- Gently release your ankle and roll over onto your left side.
- Inhale and repeat your stretch on the other side.
- To finish, bring both knees back to the center and relax in the supine position.
- Roll over onto your hands and knees, entering into the tabletop position.

Tabletop Arm and Leg Extensions

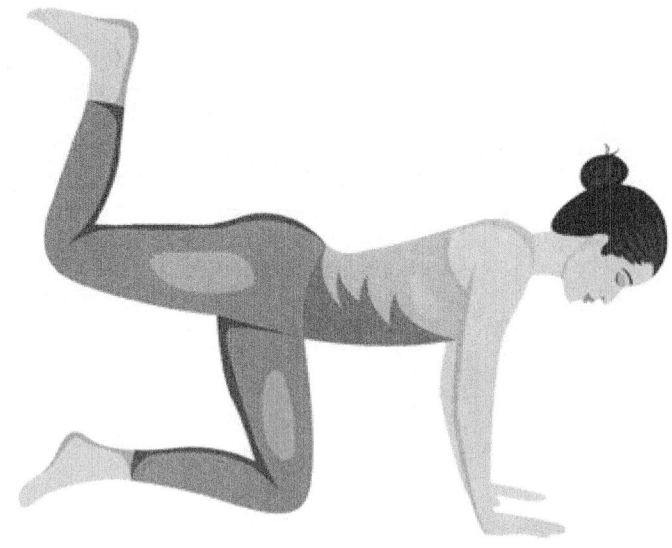

- From your tabletop position, ensure your wrists are under your shoulders and knees under your hips.
- Inhale deeply, and as you exhale, engage your core muscles.
- On your next inhale, extend your right leg straight back, keeping it parallel to the floor.
- As you extend the leg, bend your right knee, flexing your foot.
- Draw focus to your breath and maintain balance through your core.
- Hold this position and if you can, extend your left arm out straight in front of you.
- Keep your hips and shoulders square to the mat, avoiding any rotation.
- Hold this position for 5 full breath cycles, maintaining a strong and steady posture.
- With each inhale, imagine lengthening through your extended limbs.
- With each exhale, deepen your core engagement for stability.
- To release, slowly lower your extended leg and arm (if lifted) back to the starting position on an exhale.
- Repeat on the other side, extending your left leg and optionally lifting your right arm.
- Come to your center by returning to the tabletop position and rolling over onto your back.

Cool-Down Movements

Supine Knee-to-Chest Pose

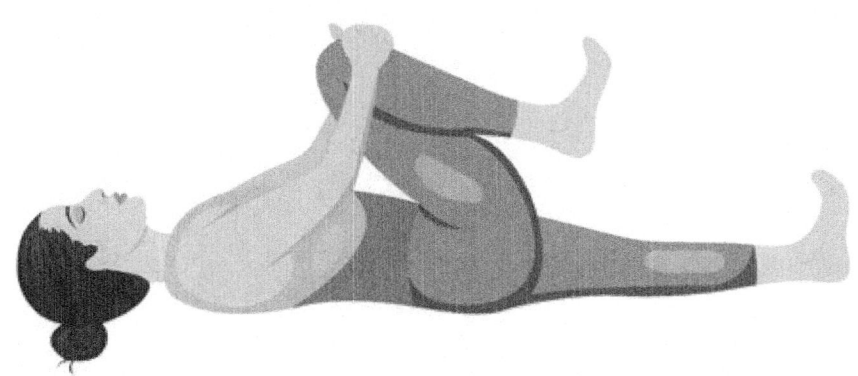

- From your supine position (lying on your back), extend both legs flat on the mat.
- Keep your feet in a neutral or toes-up flexed position.
- Inhale deeply, and as you exhale, bend your right knee and draw it towards your chest.
- Clasp your hands around your right shin or behind your thigh, whichever is more comfortable.
- Draw focus to your breath and the stretch in your right hip and lower back.
- Keep your left leg extended on the mat, pressing the back of your left thigh down.
- Gently pull your right knee closer to your chest, but avoid straining.
- Relax your shoulders and neck, keeping your head resting on the mat.
- Hold this pose for 10 full breath cycles, allowing the stretch to deepen with each exhale.
- To intensify the stretch, you can slightly lift your head and neck towards your knee.
- After 10 breaths, slowly release your right leg back to the mat.
- Repeat the sequence with your left leg, bending the left knee and drawing it to the chest.
- To finish, extend both legs on the mat and take a moment to notice the difference between sides.

Legs Up the Wall Pose/Waterfall pose

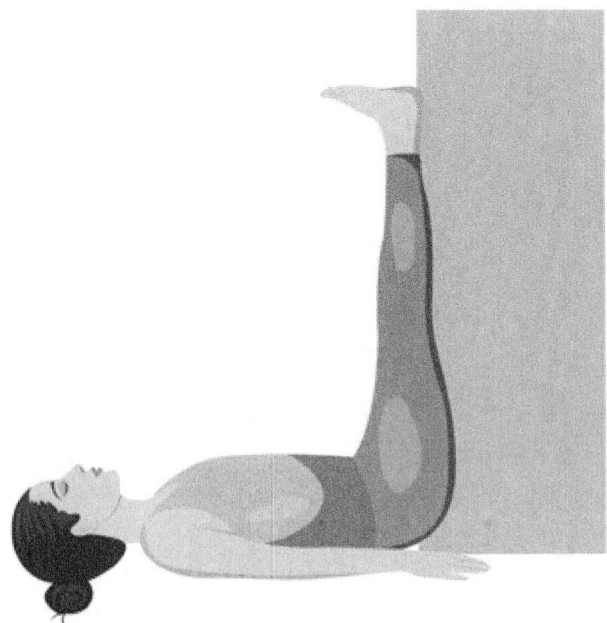

- Begin by sitting sideways close to a wall, with your hip touching the wall.
- Inhale deeply, and as you exhale, swing your legs up the wall as you lower your upper body to the floor.
- Adjust your position so your buttocks are as close to the wall as comfortable, legs extended vertically.
- Draw focus to your breath and the sensation of letting gravity do the work.
- Rest your arms by your sides, palms facing up for a relaxed position.
- Allow your legs to relax, imagining tension draining down through your body.
- If comfortable, you can slightly bend your knees to ease any hamstring tightness.
- Hold this pose for 15 full breath cycles, or longer if desired for deeper relaxation.
- With each inhale, feel your spine lengthening; with each exhale, let your body settle deeper.
- Keep your gaze soft or close your eyes to enhance the calming effect.
- To release, bend your knees and slowly roll to your side before sitting up.
- Take a moment in a seated position to notice the effects of the inversion.

Supine One-Legged Twist

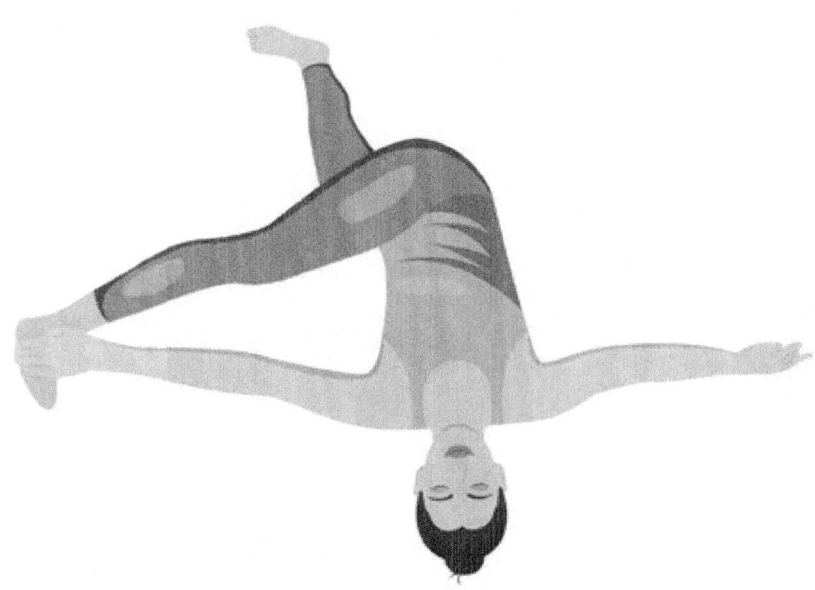

- From your supine position (lying on your back), extend both legs flat on the mat.
- Inhale deeply, and as you exhale, slide your left leg out to the right side crossing it over your body.
- If you can, reach for your left foot with your right hand. Alternatively, hold on to your leg at the calf, behind your knee, or thigh.
- Flatten your shoulders into the mat, extending your left arm out to your side in a t-position.
- Gaze over your right shoulder, drawing focus to your breath and the rotation in your spine.
- Hold this pose for 10 full breath cycles, allowing the twist to deepen with each exhale.
- Keep your right hand on your extended left leg, providing gentle pressure.
- With each inhale, lengthen your spine; with each exhale, settle deeper into the twist.
- To release, slowly unwind on an inhale, bringing your leg back to the center.
- Repeat on the other side.
- Finish by hugging both knees to your chest, then extending both legs on the mat.

SOMATIC YOGA FOR WEIGHT LOSS

Corpse Pose (Savasana)

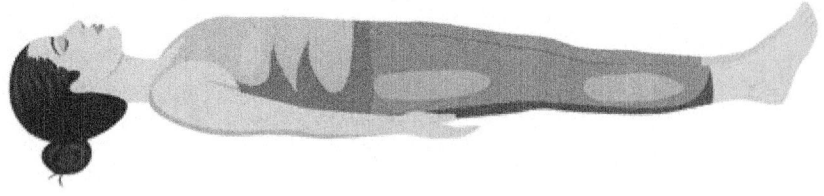

- From your supine position (lying on your back), extend your legs fully on the mat.
- Allow your feet to fall open naturally to the sides.
- Place your arms alongside your body, palms facing up.
- Inhale deeply, and as you exhale, consciously relax every part of your body.
- Draw focus to your breath, allowing it to become slow and natural.
- Systematically relax each part of your body, starting from your toes and moving up to the crown of your head.
- Let your eyes gently close and relax your facial muscles.
- Allow your body to feel heavy, sinking into the mat.
- Stay in this pose for 10 breath counts so that you can begin your guided body scan.

Guided Body Scan with Flex and Relax

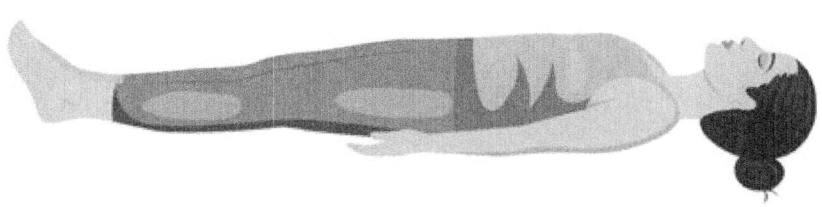

- From your supine position (lying on your back), extend your legs fully on the mat.
- Allow your arms to rest alongside your body, palms facing up.
- Inhale deeply, and as you exhale, settle into the mat.
- Draw focus to your breath, allowing it to become slow and natural.
- Begin the body scan at your feet, inhale, and flex your toes and feet.
- Exhale and completely relax them.
- Move up to your calves and thighs, inhale, and tighten these muscles.
- Exhale and release, feeling them melt into the mat.
- Continue this pattern with your glutes, abdomen, and chest:
- Inhale to engage, exhale to fully relax.
- Move to your hands and arms:
- Inhale to make fists and tense your arms.
- Exhale to release, letting your arms feel heavy.
- Focus on your shoulders and neck:
- Inhale to shrug your shoulders towards your ears.
- Exhale to drop them away, releasing all tension.
- Finally, tense and relax your facial muscles:
- Inhale to scrunch your face.
- Exhale to smooth out all lines, relaxing completely.
- Spend a few minutes in complete stillness, enjoying the deep relaxation.
- To exit, slowly wiggle your fingers and toes, then stretch gently.
- Roll to your right side and pause before slowly sitting up.

These cool-down movements help integrate the effects of your practice, promoting deep relaxation and a sense of renewal.

We will now go over specific routines designed to address stress, anxiety, and trauma. Remember that you must listen to your body and modify any pose that causes you discomfort or pain.

Access to Your Gifts

Sometimes we can become so wrapped up in linear progress that we forget about our starting point. To stay on track and ensure your somatic yoga journey is one that is peaceful, growth-oriented, and yields maximum effectiveness, we've put together two free gifts.

1. A journal that allows you to track your somatic journey, noting integral insights into your emotional and psychological state. This journal provides you with inspiration to move forward in your journey, and gives you a space to set your intentions for each workout.
2. Access to a video course that shows you how to complete your somatic movements with proper form to enhance your somatic experience.

To access your gifts, simply scan the QR code below.

Remember that consistency is key in somatic yoga practice. Try to incorporate these routines into your daily life, even if it is just for a few minutes each day. Over time, you will notice improvements in your stress levels, anxiety symptoms, and overall sense of well-being.

As always, listen to your body and respect its limits. If any movement causes pain or significant discomfort, ease off or skip it entirely. The goal is to create a safe, nurturing experience for yourself.

Routine 1: Quick Stress-Relief (10-15 minutes)

This routine is perfect for those moments when you need a quick reset during a busy day.

1. **Cat-Cow Pose** (1-2 minutes): Gently flow between arching and rounding your spine, syncing movement with breath.
2. **Pelvic Tilts** (1-2 minutes): Lying on your back, gently tilt your pelvis forward and back.
3. **Somatic Twists** (2-3 minutes): Lying on your back, let your knees fall gently from side to side.
4. **Seated Forward Fold with Rocking** (2-3 minutes): Fold forward gently and rock side to side.
5. **Seated Cat-Cow** (1-2 minutes): Recreate the Cat-Cow motion while seated.
6. **Guided Body Scan** (3-5 minutes): Close with a brief body scan, releasing tension as you go.

Routine 2: Anxiety-Calming Practice (20-30 minutes)

This routine focuses on grounding and releasing tension often associated with anxiety.

1. **Dynamic Child's Pose with arm reaches** (2-3 minutes): Move slowly, focusing on your breath.
2. **Tabletop Arm and Leg Extensions** (3-4 minutes): Move deliberately, emphasizing stability.
3. **Somatic Bridge Pose** (3-4 minutes): Focus on the sensation of your spine rolling up and down.
4. **Reclined Butterfly Pose** (3-4 minutes): Allow your knees to gently fall open and closed.
5. **Standing Pelvic Tilts** (2-3 minutes): Feel how this movement affects your whole body.
6. **Gentle Standing Twists** (2-3 minutes): Move slowly, synchronizing breath with movement.
7. **Legs Up the Wall Pose** (5-7 minutes): Let gravity help you release tension.
8. **Corpse Pose** (5 minutes): Focus on your breath and the feeling of being supported by the ground.

Routine 3: Trauma-Informed Practice (30-40 minutes)

This gentle routine is designed to help you feel safe in your body.

1. **Constructive Rest Position** (5 minutes): Begin by simply resting and breathing.
2. **Pelvic Clock** (3-4 minutes): Move slowly, exploring the range of motion in your pelvis.
3. **Somatic Shoulder Shrugs** (2-3 minutes): Focus on the sensation of tension release.
4. **Seated Arm Circles** (2-3 minutes): Move slowly, noticing how your shoulders and chest feel.
5. **Seated Cat-Cow** (3-4 minutes): Sync your movement with your breath.
6. **Seated Side Bend** (2-3 minutes on each side): Move gently, respecting your body's limits.
7. **Somatic Chest Opener** (3-4 minutes): Focus on opening and softening.
8. **Child's Pose with Arm Walks** (3-4 minutes): Move at your own pace, focusing on feeling grounded.
9. **Legs Up the Wall Pose** (5-7 minutes): Allow yourself to fully relax into this restorative pose.
10. **Guided Body Scan with Flex and Relax** (5-7 minutes): End with this relaxation technique, fostering a sense of safety in your body.

Routine 4: Morning Energizer (15-20 minutes)

This routine is designed to gently wake up your body and mind, setting a positive tone for the day.

1. **Spinal Rolls** (2-3 minutes): Start seated or standing, and slowly roll your spine up and down.
2. **Dynamic Warrior I** (2-3 minutes on each side): Move in and out of the pose, syncing with your breath.
3. **Somatic Sunbird Pose** (2-3 minutes): On hands and knees, extend and flex limbs alternately.
4. **Standing Pelvic Tilts** (2 minutes): Awaken your core with gentle pelvic movements.
5. **Dynamic Tree Pose** (1-2 minutes on each side): Practice balance while gently swaying.
6. **Somatic Forward Fold** (2-3 minutes): Bend forward and roll up slowly, focusing on each vertebra.

> SOMATIC YOGA FOR WEIGHT LOSS

7. **Chair Pose with Arm Waves** (2 minutes): Energize your whole body with this dynamic pose.
8. **Seated Cat-Cow** (2 minutes): End with gentle spinal flexion and extension.

Finish with a brief moment of seated meditation, setting an intention for your day.

Routine 5: Evening Wind-Down (25-30 minutes)

This routine helps release the tension of the day and prepare your body and mind for restful sleep.

1. **Gentle Neck Rolls** (2 minutes): Release upper body tension with slow, mindful movements.
2. **Somatic Shoulder Bridge** (3-4 minutes): Gently lift and lower your hips, focusing on the sensation.
3. **Supine Psoas Release** (3-4 minutes): Lying on your back, gently rock your bent knees side to side.
4. **Reclined Spinal Twist** (2-3 minutes on each side): Move slowly in and out of the twist.
5. **Somatic Wave** (3-4 minutes): Lying on your back, creates a wave-like motion through your spine.
6. **Sphinx Pose** (2-3 minutes): Gently lift your chest, focusing on relaxing your lower back.
7. **Child's Pose with Arm Walks** (3-4 minutes): Let your body settle into this restful pose.
8. **Legs Up the Wall Pose** (5-7 minutes): Allow gravity to help drain tension from your legs.
9. **Corpse Pose** (5 minutes): End with complete relaxation, preparing your body for sleep.

Conclude with a body scan, consciously releasing any remaining tension.

General tips for proper form and alignment

- **Breath awareness**: Always coordinate your movements with your breath to enhance the mind-body connection and promote relaxation.
- **Gentle approach**: Move slowly and mindfully. The goal is to release tension, not create it.
- **Body scanning**: Before each pose, take a moment to scan your body. This helps you identify areas of tension and adjust accordingly.
- **Use props**: Do not hesitate to use pillows, blankets, or yoga blocks to support your body. Props can help you find comfort and proper alignment in poses.
- **Respect your limits**: Never push through pain. If a pose causes discomfort, try a modification or skip it entirely.
- **Quality over quantity**: Focus on the quality of your movement and breath rather than how long you hold a pose or how many repetitions you do.
- **Symmetry**: When practicing poses that work one side of the body, always balance by practicing on the other side as well.

SOMATIC YOGA FOR WEIGHT LOSS

Chapter 4

MANAGING ANXIETY WITH SOMATIC YOGA

Anxiety can make your life a really challenging journey, but somatic yoga offers powerful tools to navigate its turbulent waters. We will now teach you how to understand and manage it through gentle, mindful practices that honor the wisdom of your body.

Understanding Anxiety and Its Triggers

Anxiety is our body's ancient alarm system, a vigilant guardian that has been with us since our earliest days as a species. Imagine our distant ancestors, navigating a world fraught with dangers—predators lurking in shadows, uncertain food sources, and rival tribes. In this context, anxiety wasn't just useful. It was essential for survival.

This innate mechanism primes us for action, sharpening our senses and readying our bodies to face potential threats. It's the feeling that made our ancestors pause before entering an unfamiliar cave or scan the horizon for signs of danger. In many ways, anxiety is a gift from our evolutionary past, a tool that helped ensure our species' survival.

Our world has changed dramatically, yet our anxiety response remains largely the same. In our modern lives, we rarely face immediate physical dangers. Instead, we worry about job interviews, social interactions, or financial pressures. Our body, however, can't always distinguish between a looming deadline and a prowling predator. It reacts to perceived threats with the same urgency, flooding our system with stress hormones and triggering that familiar feeling of unease.

Anxiety becomes problematic when this response is overactive or misaligned with actual threats. It's like having an overly sensitive smoke alarm that blares at the slightest hint of steam from your shower. The intention is good—to keep you safe—but the execution can be disruptive and distressing.

Understanding anxiety means recognizing it as a normal, even beneficial part of the human experience. It's not about eliminating anxiety entirely, but rather about calibrating our response to match the realities of our modern world. By doing so, we can harness anxiety's protective power while preventing it from overwhelming our daily lives.

Physiological Symptoms	Psychological Symptoms
• Increased heart rate and rapid breathing	• Racing thoughts or difficulty concentrating
• Muscle tension, especially in the neck, shoulders, and jaw	• Excessive worry about future events
• Digestive discomfort	• Feelings of dread or impending doom
• Sweating or chills	• Irritability or mood swings
• Fatigue or restlessness	

Anxiety can have various triggers:

- Major life changes or transitions
- Work or financial stress
- Relationship difficulties
- Health concerns
- Past traumas or phobias
- Perfectionism or self-criticism

Somatic yoga can help manage them by:

- Increasing body awareness, allowing you to recognize anxiety symptoms early
- Promoting relaxation through gentle movement and breath work
- Releasing physical tension that can exacerbate anxiety
- Cultivating a sense of grounding and present-moment focus
- Developing self-compassion and acceptance

By regularly practicing somatic yoga, you can create a buffer against anxiety triggers, making them less likely to overwhelm you.

Somatic Yoga Poses for Anxiety Relief

This routine is designed to gently release tension and promote a sense of calm. Remember, the goal is not to achieve a perfect pose, but to listen to your body and move in a way that feels supportive.

1. **Constructive Rest Position** (5 minutes): This gentle position is a cornerstone of somatic practices. As you lie there, feel the weight of your body sinking into the floor. Notice how your breath moves your hands—the hand on your belly should rise and fall more noticeably than the one on your chest. This indicates diaphragmatic breathing, which can help activate the body's relaxation response. Allow your thoughts to come and go without judgment, always returning your focus to the breath. This practice helps reset your nervous system and cultivates body awareness.
2. **Pelvic Clock** (3-4 minutes): The pelvis is often called the body's center of gravity. This exercise increases awareness and mobility in this crucial area. As you tilt your pelvis to different "hours," pay attention to how the movement affects your lower back, hips, and abdomen. Move slowly, exploring any areas of tightness or discomfort. You might notice that some directions feel easier than others - this is normal and provides valuable information about your body's patterns. The pelvic clock can help alleviate lower back tension and improve overall posture.
3. **Somatic Cat-Cow** (3-4 minutes): This variation on the classic yoga pose emphasizes slow, mindful movement. As you arch your back (Cow), inhale and feel the front of your body expanding. As you round your spine (Cat), exhale and sense the stretch across your back. Pay attention to how each vertebra moves, imagining your spine as a string of pearls rolling one bead at a time. This exercise promotes spinal flexibility and can help release tension in the back and neck.

SOMATIC YOGA FOR WEIGHT LOSS

4. **Child's Pose with Arm Reaches** (3-4 minutes): Child's Pose is deeply restorative, and adding arm reaches enhances its benefits. As you walk your hands to each side, notice the stretch along your side body, from your fingertips all the way to your hips. This movement can help release tension in the often-neglected lateral body, improving overall flexibility. Pay attention to how your breath moves into the stretched side, allowing it to create more space.

5. **Seated Forward Fold with Rocking** (3-4 minutes): This variation adds a gentle, soothing motion to a classic stretch. As you fold forward, don't worry about how far you can reach - focus instead on the sensation of the stretch and the rocking movement. The rocking can help release tension in the lower back and hamstrings. Notice how your breath changes as you move, and how the stretch might feel different on each side as you rock.

6. **Standing Mountain Pose with Body Scan** (3-4 minutes): Mountain Pose is about finding stability and alignment. As you scan your body, pay attention to areas of tension or imbalance. Are you putting more weight on one foot? Are your shoulders creeping up towards your ears? Use this awareness to make subtle adjustments. This practice improves posture and body awareness, helping you carry these benefits into your daily activities.

Each of these exercises combines movement, breath awareness, and mindfulness to promote relaxation and body awareness. Together, they form a holistic practice that addresses different areas of the body and various aspects of somatic experience.

Here is a table providing some ways to alter these poses depending on various levels of pain.

Pose	Mild discomfort	Moderate pain	Severe pain
Constructive Rest Position	Place a folded blanket under your head or knees.	Bend knees and place feet on a chair or elevated surface.	Practice in bed with pillows supporting your head and knees.
Pelvic Clock	Use a folded blanket under your hips.	Perform seated in a chair, focusing on subtle movements.	Visualize the movement without physically doing it.
Somatic Cat-Cow	Place a folded blanket under your knees.	Perform seated in a chair, focusing on spinal flexion and extension.	Practice standing, using a wall or countertop for support.
Child's Pose with Arm Reaches	Place a bolster or folded blanket under your torso.	Perform seated in a chair, reaching arms to either side.	Practice standing forward bend with gentle arm swings.
Seated Forward Fold with Rocking	Sit on a folded blanket to elevate your hips.	Perform seated in a chair, gently folding forward.	Practice standing, hands resting on a chair or countertop
Standing Mountain Pose with Body Scan	Stand with your back against a wall for support.	Perform seated in a chair with feet flat on the floor.	Practice lying down, and scanning your body in a comfortable position.

Pose	Mild discomfort	Moderate pain	Severe pain
Gentle Standing Twists	Keep feet wider apart for better stability.	Perform seated in a chair, gently twisting to each side.	Practice lying on your back, allowing your knees to fall gently from side to side.
Legs Up the Wall Pose	Place a folded blanket under your hips.	Use a chair or bed, resting your legs on an elevated surface.	Lie on your back with knees bent, and feet flat on the floor.

Finally, here are some tips to adjust your alignment during the pose.

Pose	Mild discomfort
Constructive Rest Position	Ensure your lower back is neither pressed into the floor nor excessively arched. There should be a natural, gentle curve.
Pelvic Clock	Keep your movements small and controlled. Quality of movement is more important than quantity.
Somatic Cat-Cow	Keep your neck in line with your spine, neither dropping nor lifting excessively.
Child's Pose with Arm Reaches	Keep your hips pressing back towards your heels as you reach, maintaining length in your spine.
Seated Forward Fold with Rocking	Bend your knees as much as needed to keep your back straight. Focus on hinging at the hips rather than rounding the spine.
Standing Mountain Pose with Body Scan	Distribute your weight evenly across both feet. Imagine a line of energy running from the crown of your head through your spine and down to your feet.
Gentle Standing Twists	Keep your hips facing forward as you twist, initiating the movement from your core.
Legs Up the Wall Pose	Position your sitting bones as close to the wall as is comfortable. If your hamstrings are tight, move further away from the wall.

Remember, the most important alignment in somatic yoga is the one that feels right for your body. These practices are about developing body awareness and finding what works for you. If you are unsure about a pose or experience persistent pain, it is always best to consult with a qualified yoga instructor or healthcare professional.

Breathing Techniques for Anxiety Management

The breath is a powerful tool for managing anxiety. When we are anxious, our breathing often becomes shallow and rapid. By consciously changing our breath, we can signal to our nervous system that it is safe to relax.

Square Breathing

Visualize tracing a square as you breathe:

- Inhale for 4 counts (top of the square)
- Hold for 4 counts (right side of the square)
- Exhale for 4 counts (bottom of the square)
- Hold for 4 counts (left side of the square)
- Repeat for 5-10 cycles.

4-7-8 Breath

- Inhale quietly through your nose for 4 counts
- Hold your breath for 7 counts
- Exhale completely through your mouth for 8 counts
- Repeat 4 times.

Belly Breathing

Place one hand on your belly and one on your chest.

- Inhale deeply through your nose, feeling your belly expand
- Exhale slowly through your mouth, feeling your belly contract
- Practice for 5-10 minutes.

The connection between breath and anxiety lies in its effect on our autonomic nervous system. Deep, slow breathing activates the parasympathetic nervous system, our body's "rest and digest" mode. This counteracts the sympathetic "fight or flight" response triggered by anxiety.

Remember, like any skill, these techniques become more effective with regular practice. Try incorporating them into your daily routine, not just when you are feeling anxious.

By combining somatic yoga poses with mindful breathing techniques, you are building a powerful toolkit for managing anxiety. As you continue your practice, you may find that not only do you handle anxious moments better, but you also experience fewer of them overall.

Chapter 5

STRESS RELIEF THROUGH SOMATIC YOGA

Along with anxiety, stress has now become a troublesome companion for many. This chapter explores how somatic yoga can be a powerful ally in managing stress, helping you cultivate a sense of calm and balance in your daily life.

Identifying Stressors in Your Life

Firstly, you need to spot the sources of stress in your life to cope with them efficiently. Stressors can be external (from your environment) or internal (from your thoughts and beliefs).

Common External Stressors	Common Internal Stressors
Work pressures and deadlines	Perfectionism or unrealistic expectations
Financial concerns	Negative self-talk
Relationship difficulties	Worry about future events
Major life changes (moving, job loss, etc.)	Unresolved past traumas
Environmental factors (noise, crowding	Fear of failure or success

Here are some strategies for recognizing them:

- Keep a stress journal: Note when you feel stressed, what triggered it, and how you responded.

SOMATIC YOGA FOR WEIGHT LOSS

- Body awareness practice: Regularly check in with your body. Where do you hold tension?
- Emotion tracking: Notice which emotions arise most frequently and in what situations.
- Lifestyle audit: Examine your daily routines. Are there consistent sources of stress?

Remember, identifying these stressors is not about getting rid of them, but about understanding them. This awareness will allow you to respond more skillfully to stress when it arises.

Somatic Yoga for Relaxation

The following routine is designed to release tension and promote relaxation. As always, listen to your body and modify as needed.

1. Constructive Rest Position (5 minutes)

Lie on your back, knees bent, feet flat on the floor. Place one hand on your belly and one on your chest.

Modification	Alignment Tip
Use pillows under the knees and head for comfort.	Ensure your lower back has a natural curve, neither pressed to the floor nor overly arched.

2. Somatic Psoas Release (3-4 minutes on each side)

Lie on your back, one leg extended, the other knee bent with the foot flat. Gently rock the bent knee side to side.

Modification	Alignment Tip
If hip discomfort arises, place a folded blanket under the hip of the bent leg.	Keep your lower back stable as you move the leg.

3. Seated Spinal Waves (3-4 minutes)

Sit comfortably, imagining your spine as a wave. Gently roll forward and back, side to side.

Modification	Alignment Tip
Practice in a chair if sitting on the floor is uncomfortable.	Initiate the movement from your tailbone, letting it ripple up your spine.

4. **Standing Forward Bend with Arm Swings (3-4 minutes)**

Stand with feet hip-width apart. Bend forward, letting your arms and head hang heavy. Gently swing arms from side to side

Modification	Alignment Tip
Bend your knees generously to protect your lower back.	Hinge from your hips rather than rounding your back.

5. **Gentle Seated Twist (2-3 minutes on each side)**

Sit comfortably, placing one hand behind you and the other on the opposite knee. Gently twist, initiating from your core.

Modification	Alignment Tip
Practice in a chair if floor sitting is difficult.	Keep your spine long as you twist, imagining growing taller.

6. **Legs Up the Wall (5-7 minutes)**

Lie on your back with your legs extended up a wall.

Modification	Alignment Tip
If this is uncomfortable, try lying on your back with your knees bent, and your feet flat on the floor.	Scoot your sitting bones as close to the wall as is comfortable.

Meditation and Mindfulness Practices

Integrating meditation and mindfulness with somatic yoga can deepen your stress relief practice. These techniques help cultivate present-moment awareness and a non-judgmental attitude toward our experiences.

Here is a non-exhaustive list of the benefits of meditation and mindfulness for stress relief:

- Reduces rumination and worry
- Improves emotional regulation
- Enhances body awareness
- Promotes relaxation response
- Increases resilience to stress

Meditation Technique: Body Scan Meditation

1. Lie comfortably on your back or sit in a supported position.
2. Close your eyes and take a few deep breaths to center yourself.
3. Begin at your toes, bringing your full attention to the sensations there.
4. Slowly move your attention up your body - feet, ankles, calves, knees, and so on.
5. At each area, notice any sensations without trying to change them.
6. If you notice tension, breathe into that area and imagine it softening.
7. Continue until you've scanned your entire body.

Practice for 10-15 minutes daily, gradually increasing the duration as you become more comfortable.

Mindfulness Exercise: STOP Technique

This quick mindfulness practice can be done anywhere, anytime you feel stressed:

S - Stop what you are doing

T - Take a breath

O - Observe your thoughts, feelings, and bodily sensations

P - Proceed with awareness

Integrating these practices with your somatic yoga routine can create a powerful stress management toolkit. Remember, consistency is key. Even a few minutes of practice each day can lead to significant benefits over time.

As you explore these techniques, be patient and compassionate with yourself. Stress relief is a skill that develops with practice.

SOMATIC YOGA FOR WEIGHT LOSS

Chapter 6

TRAUMA RELEASE WITH SOMATIC YOGA

Trauma can leave lasting imprints on both our minds and bodies. Somatic yoga offers a gentle, body-centered approach to processing and releasing trauma. This chapter introduces specific practices designed to help you reconnect with your body and release stored tension in a safe, controlled manner.

Routine

Remember, when working with trauma, it's crucial to move slowly and respect your body's boundaries. If any practice feels overwhelming, pause and return to a neutral, grounding position.

1. **Grounding Practice: Seated Mountain Pose (5 minutes)**

Sit comfortably on the floor or in a chair. Focus on feeling the points of contact between your body and the surface beneath you.

Modification	Alignment Tip
If sitting is uncomfortable, try lying down.	Imagine a line of energy extending from the base of your spine through the crown of your head.

SOMATIC YOGA FOR WEIGHT LOSS

2. Gentle Spinal Flexion and Extension (3-4 minutes)

From a seated position, gently round your spine forward on an exhale, then arch it back on an inhale.

Modification	Alignment Tip
If you have back pain, keep the movements very small.	Move slowly, focusing on articulating each vertebra.

3. Arm Swings with Sound (3-4 minutes)

Stand with feet hip-width apart. Swing your arms forward and up on an inhale, making a gentle "ha" sound as you exhale and swing them back down.

Modification	Alignment Tip
Practice seated if standing is challenging.	Let your knees soften as you swing to avoid locking your joints.

4. Slow Neck Rolls (2-3 minutes)

Gently roll your head in a half-circle from one shoulder to the other, keeping the back of your neck long.

Modification	Alignment Tip
If you experience dizziness, keep your gaze fixed on a point in front of you.	Imagine your head being gently pulled upward as you roll, creating space in your neck.

5. Butterfly Pose with Forward Fold (4-5 minutes)

Sit with the soles of your feet together, knees out to the sides. Gently fold forward, allowing your spine to round.

Modification	Alignment Tip
Sit on a cushion to elevate your hips if your knees are higher than your hips.	Focus on relaxing your inner thighs and groin area.

6. **Reclined Bound Angle Pose (5-7 minutes)**

Lie on your back with the soles of your feet together, knees out to the sides. Place one hand on your belly and one on your heart.

Modification	Alignment Tip
Support your knees with pillows if you feel any strain in your hips or groin.	Allow your lower back to maintain its natural curve.

Additional Somatic Practices for Trauma Release

- **Shaking Practice (2-3 minutes)**

Stand with knees slightly bent. Begin gently shaking your body, starting from your feet and moving upward. Allow your arms to flop loosely.

This practice can help release tension and stuck energy in the body.

- **Self-Holding (5 minutes)**

Place one hand on your forehead and one on your heart. Focus on your breath and the warmth of your hands.

This simple practice can help you feel safe and contained.

- **Tension and Release (3-4 minutes)**

Progressively tense and then relax different muscle groups in your body. Start with your feet and move upward.

This practice increases body awareness and promotes relaxation.

- **Mindful Walking (5-10 minutes)**

Walk slowly, paying close attention to the sensation of your feet touching the ground. Coordinate your breath with your steps.

This practice combines movement, breath awareness, and grounding.

- **Humming (2-3 minutes)**

Take a deep breath in, then hum on the exhale. Notice the vibration in your chest and throat.

Humming can help activate the vagus nerve, promoting relaxation.

When working with traumas, there are some safeguards that you should always keep in mind.

- Always prioritize feeling safe. If a practice does not feel right, it is okay to stop or modify.
- Move slowly and mindfully. Trauma release is not about pushing your limits.
- Stay present. If you notice yourself dissociating, try a grounding practice like feeling your feet on the floor.
- Be patient and compassionate with yourself. Healing is a process and every small step counts.
- Consider working with a trauma-informed yoga teacher or therapist for personalized guidance.

Integrating these somatic yoga practices into your routine can support your journey of trauma release. However, they are not a substitute for professional mental health care. If you are dealing with significant trauma, please seek support from a qualified mental health professional.

Remember, you are not alone in this journey. Many have found healing through somatic practices, and with patience and persistence, you can too. Trust in your body's innate wisdom and capacity for healing.

Chapter 7

28-DAY SOMATIC YOGA PLAN

We will begin this chapter with some routines and techniques to implement into a 28-day plan to improve your physical and mental well-being.

Routines and techniques

Anxiety Relief Routine (15-20 minutes)

1. **Constructive Rest Position (3-4 minutes)**
   Lie on your back, knees bent, feet flat on the floor. Place one hand on your belly and one on your chest.

2. **Pelvic Clock (2-3 minutes)**
   Remaining in the same position, gently tilt your pelvis in different "clock" directions.

3. **Somatic Cat-Cow (3-4 minutes)**
   On hands and knees, alternate between arching and rounding your spine, moving slowly with your breath.

4. **Child's Pose with Arm Reaches (2-3 minutes)**
   From Child's Pose, slowly walk your hands to one side, then the other.

5. **Seated Forward Fold with Rocking (2-3 minutes)**
   Sit with legs extended. Fold forward gently, allowing your upper body to rock side to side.

6. **Standing Mountain Pose with Body Scan (2-3 minutes)**
   Stand tall, feet hip-width apart. Slowly scan your body from feet to head, releasing tension.

7. **Legs Up the Wall Pose (3-4 minutes)**
   Lie on your back with your legs extended up a wall.

Stress Relief Routine (15-20 minutes)

1. **Constructive Rest Position (3-4 minutes)**
   As described above.

2. **Somatic Psoas Release (3-4 minutes on each side)**
   Lie on your back, one leg extended, the other knee bent with the foot flat. Gently rock the bent knee side to side.

3. **Seated Spinal Waves (3-4 minutes)**
   Sit comfortably, imagining your spine as a wave. Gently roll forward and back, side to side.

4. **Standing Forward Bend with Arm Swings (3-4 minutes)**
   Stand with feet hip-width apart. Bend forward, letting your arms and head hang heavy. Gently swing arms from side to side.

5. **Gentle Seated Twist (2-3 minutes on each side)**
   Sit comfortably, placing one hand behind you and the other on the opposite knee. Gently twist, initiating from your core.

6. **Legs Up the Wall (3-4 minutes)**
   As described above.

Trauma Release Routine (15 to 20 minutes)

1. **Grounding Practice: Seated Mountain Pose (3 4 minutes)**
   Sit comfortably, focusing on feeling the points of contact between your body and the surface beneath you.

2. **Gentle Spinal Flexion and Extension (3-4 minutes)**
   From a seated position, gently round your spine forward on an exhale, then arch it back on an inhale.

3. **Arm Swings with Sound (2-3 minutes)**
   Stand with feet hip-width apart. Swing your arms forward and up on an inhale, making a gentle "ha" sound as you exhale and swing them back down.

4. **Slow Neck Rolls (2-3 minutes)**
   Gently roll your head in a half-circle from one shoulder to the other, keeping the back of your neck long.

5. **Butterfly Pose with Forward Fold (3-4 minutes)**
   Sit with the soles of your feet together, knees out to the sides. Gently fold forward, allowing your spine to round.

6. **Reclined Bound Angle Pose (4-5 minutes)**
   Lie on your back with the soles of your feet together, knees out to the sides. Place one hand on your belly and one on your heart.

Breathing Techniques

1. **Square Breathing (3-5 minutes)**
   Visualize tracing a square as you breathe: Inhale for 4 counts, hold for 4, exhale for 4, hold for 4. Repeat.

2. **4-7-8 Breath (3-5 minutes)**
   Inhale for 4 counts, hold for 7, exhale for 8. Repeat.

3. **Belly Breathing (5-10 minutes)**
   Place one hand on your belly. Inhale deeply through your nose, feeling your belly expand. Exhale slowly through your mouth, feeling your belly contract.

Mindfulness Practices

1. Body Scan Meditation (10-15 minutes)
Lie comfortably. Bring attention to each part of your body sequentially from your toes to head, noticing sensations without judgment.

2. Mindful Walking (5-10 minutes)
Walk slowly, paying close attention to the sensation of your feet touching the ground. Coordinate your breath with your steps.

3. STOP Technique (can be done in 1-2 minutes, practice multiple times a day)
Stop, Take a breath, Observe your thoughts/feelings/sensations, and proceed with awareness.

4. Shaking Practice (2-3 minutes)
Stand with knees slightly bent. Begin gently shaking your body, starting from your feet and moving upward.

5. Self-Holding (5 minutes)
Place one hand on your forehead and one on your heart. Focus on your breath and the warmth of your hands.

6. Tension and Release (3-4 minutes)
Progressively tense and then relax different muscle groups in your body, starting from your feet and moving upward.

28-Day Plan

This comprehensive plan integrates somatic yoga poses, breathing techniques, and mindfulness practices to help you establish a consistent routine for managing stress, anxiety, and trauma. Each week builds upon the previous one, gradually introducing new elements while reinforcing core practices.

Week 1: Foundation

Day 1:

- Morning: 5 minutes Constructive Rest Position
- Evening: 3-5 minutes Square Breathing

Day 2:

- Morning: 5 minutes Pelvic Clock
- Evening: 5 minutes Body Scan Meditation

Day 3:

- Morning: 5 minutes Somatic Cat-Cow
- Evening: 3-5 minutes 4-7-8 Breath

Day 4:

- Morning: 5 minutes Seated Spinal Waves
- Evening: 5 minutes of Mindful Walking

Day 5:

- Morning: 5 minutes Standing Mountain Pose with Body Scan
- Evening: 3-5 minutes Belly Breathing

Day 6:

- Morning: 5 minutes Gentle Standing Twists
- Evening: 5 minutes STOP Technique practice

Day 7:

- Morning: 10 minutes combining favorite poses from the week
- Evening: 10 minutes reflection on the week's practice

Week 2: Building Awareness

Day 8:

- Morning: 10 minutes Constructive Rest Position + Pelvic Clock
- Evening: 5 minutes Square Breathing

Day 9:

- Morning: 10 minutes Somatic Cat-Cow + Child's Pose with Arm Reaches
- Evening: 7 minutes Body Scan Meditation

Day 10:

- Morning: 10 minutes Seated Forward Fold with Rocking + Seated Spinal Waves
- Evening: 5 minutes 4-7-8 Breath

Day 11:

- Morning: 10 minutes Standing Mountain Pose + Gentle Standing Twists
- Evening: 7 minutes of Mindful Walking

Day 12:

- Morning: 10 minutes Legs Up the Wall Pose
- Evening: 7 minutes of Belly Breathing

Day 13:

- Morning: 15 minutes combining favorite poses from the week
- Evening: 5 minutes STOP Technique practice

Day 14:

- Morning: 15 minutes gentle flow combining week's poses
- Evening: 10 minutes reflection on the week's practice

Week 3: Deepening Practice

Day 15:

- Morning: 15-minute Anxiety Relief Routine (from Chapter 4)
- Evening: 10 minutes Square Breathing + Body Scan Meditation

Day 16:

- Morning: 15-minute Stress Relief Routine (from Chapter 5)
- Evening: 10 minutes 4-7-8 Breath + Mindful Walking

Day 17:

- Morning: 15 minutes Trauma Release Routine (from Chapter 6)
- Evening: 10 minutes Belly Breathing + STOP Technique

Day 18:

- Morning: 20 minutes combining favorite poses from previous days
- Evening: 15 minutes Body Scan Meditation

Day 19:

- Morning: 20 minutes Anxiety Relief Routine
- Evening: 10 minutes Shaking Practice + Self-Holding

Day 20:

- Morning: 20 minutes Stress Relief Routine
- Evening: 10 minutes Tension and Release Practice

Day 21:

- Morning: 20 minutes Trauma Release Routine
- Evening: 15 minutes reflection on the week's practice

Week 4: Integration

Day 22:

- Morning: 25 minutes combining Anxiety and Stress Relief practices
- Evening: 15 minutes meditation of choice

Day 23:

- Morning: 25 minutes combining Stress Relief and Trauma Release practices
- Evening: 15 minutes breathing technique of choice

Day 24:

- Morning: 25 minutes combining Anxiety Relief and Trauma Release practices
- Evening: 15 minutes of mindfulness practice of choice

Day 25:

- Morning: 30 minutes creating your own routine from favorite practices
- Evening: 20 minutes Body Scan Meditation

Day 26:

- Morning: 30-minute Anxiety Relief Routine + breathing techniques
- Evening: 20 minutes Mindful Walking + STOP Technique

Day 27:

- Morning: 30-minute Stress Relief Routine + mindfulness practices
- Evening: 20 minutes Self-Holding + Tension and Release

Day 28:

- Morning: 30 minutes Trauma Release Routine + favorite practices
- Evening: 30-minute reflection on the 28-day journey

By the end of this 28-day plan, you should have a good understanding of various somatic yoga practices and how they affect you. Use this knowledge to create a personalized routine that best serves your needs going forward.

Remember, the goal is not perfection, but rather developing a sustainable practice that supports your well-being. Feel free to adjust the timing of practices to fit your schedule.

CONCLUSION: MAINTAINING YOUR SOMATIC YOGA PRACTICE

As we reach the end of our journey together, it is important to remember that this is just the beginning of your lifelong exploration of somatic yoga. The practices you have learned are tools that can support you through life's ups and downs, helping you cultivate resilience, self-awareness, and inner peace.

Continuing Your Journey

Maintaining motivation for any practice can be challenging, but the benefits of consistent somatic yoga are well worth the effort. Here are some strategies to help you stay committed:

1. **Set New Goals:**

- Establish both short-term and long-term goals for your practice.
- Make your goals SMART: Specific, Measurable, Achievable, Relevant, and Time-bound.
- Example: "I will practice somatic yoga for 20 minutes, 5 days a week, for the next month."

2. **Find Inspiration:**

- Keep a yoga journal to track your progress and insights.
- Join a community of like-minded practitioners, either in-person or online.
- Explore new somatic yoga resources, such as books, workshops, or retreats.

3. **Integrate Yoga into Daily Life:**

- Practice mini-sessions during your workday, like desk stretches or breathing exercises.
- Use everyday activities as opportunities for mindfulness, like mindful eating or walking.

- Create a dedicated space in your home for your practice, even if it is just a corner of a room.

Adapting to Life Changes

Life is constantly changing, and your yoga practice should evolve with it. Here is how you can adapt your practice to various life circumstances:

1. Aging:

- Focus on gentle, low-impact movements that maintain flexibility and balance.
- Incorporate more restorative poses and longer holds to support joint health.
- Example: John, 65, shifted from dynamic flows to slower, more deliberate movements, finding greater benefit in mindful practice.

2. Injury or Illness:

- Work with a healthcare provider or yoga therapist to modify your practice safely.
- Emphasize breathwork and meditation when physical practice is limited.
- Example: Maria, recovering from knee surgery, focused on seated and reclined poses, maintaining her practice without straining her knee.

3. Major Life Events (new job, moving, having a baby):

- Be flexible with your practice time and duration.
- Use your practice as a grounding tool during times of change.
- Example: Tom, a new father, integrated short yoga sessions into his baby's nap times, finding moments of calm in a busy new schedule.

Strategies for Staying Engaged

1. Explore different styles of yoga that complement your somatic practice.
2. Attend workshops or retreats to deepen your understanding and reignite your passion.
3. Consider becoming a yoga teacher or mentor, sharing your experience with others.

4. Use technology, like yoga apps or online classes, to vary your routine and stay motivated.

Remember, your yoga practice is uniquely yours. It is okay for it to change and evolve as you do. The most important thing is to keep showing up on your mat, even if it looks different from day to day.

As we conclude this guide, I want to express my gratitude for allowing me to be a part of your somatic yoga journey. Your commitment to self-discovery and growth is truly inspiring.

Remember, the journey of somatic yoga is ongoing. Each day brings new opportunities for growth, self-discovery, and healing. Trust in your body's wisdom, be patient with yourself, and celebrate every step of your progress, no matter how small it may seem.

Thank you for your dedication to your practice and for being a part of this somatic yoga community. May your journey continue to bring you peace, strength, and deep connection with yourself.

Namaste.

EXERCISE LIST

Cat-Cow Pose (Marjaryasana-Bitilasana) 20
Dynamic Child's Pose (Balasana) 21
Spinal Rolls. 22
Pelvic Tilts 23
Gentle Neck Rolls. 24
Core Somatic Yoga Poses. 25
Arch and Flatten. 25
Chair Pose with Arm Waves 26
Child's Pose with Arm Walks 27
Constructive Rest Position 28
Dynamic Bridge Pose 29
Dynamic Downward Dog 30
Dynamic Tree Pose 31
Dynamic Warrior I 32
Gentle Fish Pose (Matsyasana) 33
Knees to Chest Rocking 35
Leg Slides. 36
Lying Hip Release 37
Pelvic Clock 38
Quadruped Cat Stretch 39
Reclined Butterfly Pose 40
Reclined Hamstring Stretch 41
Reclined Spinal Twist 42
Seated Arm Circles 43
Seated Cat-Cow. 44
Seated Figure Four Stretch 45
Seated Forward Fold with Rocking 46
Seated Side Bend 47
Side-Lying Leg Lifts 48
Somatic Bridge Pose 49
Somatic Chest Opener 50
Somatic Cobra Pose 51
Somatic Crescent Lunge 52
Somatic Forward Fold 53
Somatic Frog Pose 54
Somatic Half-Bow Pose 55
Somatic Hip Rolls. 56
Standing Pelvic Tilts 57

Somatic Pigeon Pose 58
Somatic Plank Pose 59
Somatic Scapula Mobilization 60
Somatic Seated Twist 61
Somatic Side Stretch 62
Somatic Shoulder Bridge 63
Somatic Shoulder Shrugs 64
Somatic Sunbird Pose. 65
Somatic Twists 66
Somatic Tabletop Cat-Cow 67
Somatic Warrior II 68
Somatic Wave. 69
Sphinx Pose 70
Standing Forward Bend with Swaying 71
Supine Arm Circles. 72
Supine PSOAS Release. 73
Tabletop Arm and Leg Extensions 74
Cool-Down Movements 75
Supine Knee-to-Chest Pose 75
Legs Up the Wall Pose/Waterfall pose 76
Supine One-Legged Twist 77
Corpse Pose (Savasana) 78
Guided Body Scan with Flex and Relax 79

REFERENCES

Blanchfield, T. (2024, February 7). What to Know About Somatic Experiencing Therapy. Verywell Mind. https://www.verywellmind.com/what-is-somatic-experiencing-5204186

Courtney, D. (2022, December 5). What Is Somatic Therapy? Forbes Health. https://www.forbes.com/health/mind/somatic-therapy/#:~:text=Somatic%20therapy%2C%20sometimes%20known%20as

Eichenseher, T. (2022, February 8). What You Need to Know About Somatic Yoga. Yoga Journal. https://www.yogajournal.com/practice/somatics-yoga/

Fincham, G. W., Strauss, C., Montero-Marin, J., & Cavanagh, K. (2023). Effect of Breathwork on Stress and Mental Health: a meta-analysis of randomized-controlled Trials. Scientific Reports, 13(1). https://doi.org/10.1038/s41598-022-27247-y

Ghiur, E. C., Sachini Akuretiya, Teodora. (2023, September 11). 10 Somatic Exercises To Release Pent-Up Emotions. BetterMe Blog. https://betterme.world/articles/somatic-exercises/

Menezes, C. B., Dalpiaz, N. R., Kiesow, L. G., Sperb, W., Hertzberg, J., & Oliveira, A. A. (2015). Yoga and emotion regulation: A review of primary psychological outcomes and their physiological correlates. Psychology & Neuroscience, 8(1), 82–101. https://doi.org/10.1037/h0100353

Salamon, M. (2023, July 7). What is somatic therapy? Harvard Health. https://www.health.harvard.edu/blog/what-is-somatic-therapy-202307072951

6 Ways Somatic Movement Can Benefit Your Mind and Body. (n.d.). The Output. https://www.onepeloton.com/blog/somatic-movement/

Somatic Self Care. (n.d.). Www.hopkinsmedicine.org. https://www.hopkinsmedicine.org/office-of-well-being/connection-support/somatic-self-care

Somatic Therapy | Psychology Today. (n.d.). Www.psychologytoday.com. https://www.psychologytoday.com/intl/therapy-types/somatic-therapy

Stoddart, E.-J. (2024, February 2). What is somatic exercise and how can it boost your wellbeing? Glamour UK. https://www.glamourmagazine.co.uk/article/somatic-exercise

van de Kamp, Scheffers, M., Emck, C., Fokker, T. J., Janneke Hatzmann, Pim Cuijpers, & Beek, P. J. (2023). Body‐and movement‐oriented interventions for posttraumatic stress disorder: An updated systematic review and meta‐analysis. Journal of Traumatic Stress. https://doi.org/10.1002/jts.22968

Yoga and Somatics. (n.d.). Ekhart Yoga. https://www.ekhartyoga.com/resources/styles/yoga-and-somatics

Printed in Great Britain
by Amazon